"Yoga was originally taught and practiced as a tool for spiritual growth, as a way to integrate the spiritual self with the physical self. Its origins come from indigenous people with roots in India and Africa. Black people have a rich history of spiritual and healing practices that support health, resilience, and well-being that are compatible with yoga philosophy and practice. *Yoga in the Black Community* offers a well-documented and comprehensive overview of these practices and gives voice to the presence of Blacks within the yoga community. A must-read."

—*Gail Parker, PhD, C-IAYT, psychologist, yoga therapist educator, and author of* Restorative Yoga for Ethnic and Race-Based Stress and Trauma, *and* Transforming Ethnic and Race-Based Traumatic Stress with Yoga

"*Yoga in the Black Community* expertly weaves the culture, legacy, and history of being Black in the US with the spiritual grounding offered through yoga philosophy and practices. Charlene Muhammad and Marilyn Peppers-Citizen give shape and context to their explanations by illuminating both the African and American influence on Black culture while relating all of it to the spiritual practices of yoga. This book is a desperately needed guide to those in the Black community considering yoga as a health practice."

—*Kimberly Middleton, RN, MPH, MS, RYT500, founder and owner of Path of Compassion, LLC https://path-of-compassion.org*

"Muhammad and Peppers-Citizen are making an incredibly important contribution to our understanding of yoga, what it is, its relationship to Black communities and who it is 'for.' This ground-breaking book blows apart the stereotypes around yoga as exercise for 'other' people, to explore Black people's deep historical and cultural relationships to the practice. The authors provide evidence-based research on the positive impact of yoga on reducing violence, improving health, advancing healing in our communities, and, perhaps most importantly, they go on to show us how to create vital spaces of practice in our own communities. Part history, part guide, part clear-eyed critique of the harm Black people suffer living under racism and anti-Blackness, *Yoga in the Black Community* is a must-read for anyone committed to health and healing in Black communities."

—*Makani Themba, Chief Strategist at Higher Ground Change Strategies and author of* Making Policy, Making Change

"This is a powerfully written book that enhances interconnection with mind, body, and spirit."

—*Thomas W. Johnson, MD, MBA*

"This book is a celebration of community, vitality, joy, and health. Whether you are a committed yogi or just a seeker looking for more peace and wellness in your life, Muhammad and Peppers-Citizen are excellent companions on the mat and on the page."

—*Karen Valby, author of* The Swans of Harlem

"*Yoga in the Black Community* is an essential book for Black people who engage in yoga practice, as well as for anyone who teaches yoga in communities of color. Along with instruction about the physical and contemplative aspects of the practice, Muhammad and Peppers-Citizen acknowledge the historical, social, and spiritual context in which Black people are practicing yoga. This understanding is critical to a skillful and safe practice. This book will have a prominent place on my yoga bookshelf."

—*Tamara Jeffries, yoga teacher, writer, and former Senior Editor,* Yoga Journal

"This is a book that I will return to time after time. It delves into the historical and social challenges faced by the Black community, offering a perspective that's both thought-provoking and empowering. It has answered so many questions about the reason why yoga is not readily embraced by the Black community. It is a compelling read for anyone who wishes to make yoga and well-being spaces truly diverse and inclusive. Thank you, Marilyn and Charlene, for writing this much-needed book. It is a gift to the Black community and a vital message for all yogis who want to see the practice evolve into a truly welcoming space for everyone. A powerful read for people of all races."

—*Donna Noble, author of* Teaching Body Positive Yoga

"*Yoga in the Black Community* is a rejuvenating dive into yoga's true essence, far beyond the surface-level asana. This book is a call to reconnect with both yoga practices and rituals from our African ancestors, offering a path back to self and nature in our technology-driven world. It addresses health disparities in the Black community, presenting yoga and spiritual practices as powerful healing tools, complete with facts and recipes. This book will be a treasured resource for my studio and trainings."

—*Dana A. Smith, E-RYT500, owner of Spiritual Essence Yoga & Wellness*

YOGA IN THE
BLACK COMMUNITY

of related interest

Restorative Yoga for Ethnic and Race-Based Stress and Trauma
Gail Parker
Forewords by Octavia F. Raheem and Amy Wheeler
Illustrations by Justine Ross
ISBN 978 1 78775 185 9
eISBN 978 1 78775 186 6

Transforming Ethnic and Race-Based Traumatic Stress with Yoga
Gail Parker
Illustrations by Justine Ross
ISBN 978 1 78775 753 0
eISBN 978 1 78775 754 7

Yoga – Anticolonial Philosophy
An Action-Focused Guide to Practice
Shyam Ranganathan
ISBN 978 1 83997 876 0
eISBN 978 1 83997 877 7

YOGA
in the **BLACK**
COMMUNITY
HEALING PRACTICES
AND PRINCIPLES

Charlene Marie Muhammad
and **Marilyn Peppers-Citizen**

Forewords by Jana Long and Krishna Kaur

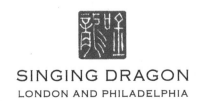

SINGING DRAGON
LONDON AND PHILADELPHIA

First published in Great Britain in 2024 by Singing Dragon,
an imprint of Jessica Kingsley Publishers
Part of John Murray Press

1

Photography by Lorenzo Wilkins and Taj Hakim Martinez

Front cover image source: Shutterstock®. The cover image is for
illustrative purposes only, and any person featuring is a model.

A CIP catalogue record for this title is available from the
British Library and the Library of Congress

ISBN 978 1 83997 862 3
eISBN 978 1 83997 863 0

Printed and bound in the United States by Integrated Books International

Jessica Kingsley Publishers' policy is to use papers that are natural,
renewable and recyclable products and made from wood grown in
sustainable forests. The logging and manufacturing processes are expected
to conform to the environmental regulations of the country of origin.

Singing Dragon
Carmelite House
50 Victoria Embankment
London EC4Y 0DZ

www.singingdragon.com

John Murray Press
Part of Hodder & Stoughton Limited
An Hachette UK Company

Dedication

We dedicate this work to the continuing healing and well-being of Black communities throughout the diaspora and everywhere else we call home.

Disclaimer

All material provided in this book is for educational purposes only. The recommendations are provided for general knowledge and are not intended to be a substitute for medical advice. Please consult with your healthcare provider to evaluate if any of these interventions are appropriate for you or your students before practicing them.

Contents

Foreword

JANA LONG, EXECUTIVE DIRECTOR, BLACK YOGA TEACHERS ALLIANCE

How I wish I had access to a book like this when I was navigating the transition from yoga practitioner to yoga teacher. *Yoga in the Black Community: Healing Practices and Principles*, by Charlene Marie Muhammad and Marilyn Peppers-Citizen, provides compelling evidence of how the healing power of yoga can bring peaceful transformation and holistic healing to Black individuals, their families, and communities.

Yoga in the Black Community: Healing Practices and Principles is both revolutionary and revelatory. It affirms what we already know deep within us—that we come from a lineage of remarkably strong and resilient people. As we reconnect with our ancestral memory, embrace nature, and honor our creative spirit, we discover enduring ways of living and being that inspire others and lead us to higher aspirations, akin to the mountaintop Dr. Martin Luther King, Jr. spoke of on the eve of his assassination when he said, "We've got some difficult days ahead. But I want you to know tonight, that we, as a people, will get to the promised land."

Muhammad and Peppers-Citizen show us how yoga, in its full expression of philosophy and practice, offers a prescription for healing the bodies, minds, hearts, and souls of Black individuals as recognized by W.E.B. DuBois. As someone who first became aware of yoga in the early 1970s, I recall the scarcity of books that focused on the physical postures of hatha yoga. Most of my readings delved into interpretations and principles of the ancient texts of Vedic culture, dating back thousands of years.

The Yoga Sutras of Patanjali have profoundly influenced my understanding of the purpose of yoga in my pursuit of spiritual development.

During that period, I longed for literature that delved deeper into the philosophical principles underlying yoga. The universal nature of yoga as a practical guide for embracing a spiritual life deeply resonated with me. Patanjali's eight-limb system, which he codified, appeared relevant and accessible to all seekers, irrespective of their race, ethnicity, culture, or religion. More recent discussions surrounding cultural appropriation and the association of Hinduism with yoga sparked fresh inquiries regarding my personal connection to the practice. Eventually, I found solace in acknowledging that "yoga" originates from the ancient Sanskrit language, signifying "union," and specifically referring to the harmonious integration of the divine aspects of human existence: body, mind, and spirit. I have no doubt that numerous ancient cultures and individuals practiced various forms of union, but the specific terminology used by them has been lost to the passage of time, whereas the term "yoga" has endured.

Yoga shares common threads with various philosophies, secular and religious doctrines, and dogmas. As more light was shed on yoga and its profound complexities, more books written, more diverse voices and narratives espousing its virtues, I became acutely aware of the lack of Black voices—our philosophers, teachers, academics, researchers, and writers. The African voice had been rendered silent, with ways of being and healing practices handed down through oral tradition rather than written word; that is, until now.

Muhammad and Peppers-Citizen have done a remarkable job of presenting evidence-based research, primarily drawing from the work of Black scholars, health professionals, and academics. This research supports the intersection of yoga and its philosophy with traditional healing practices in the Black community, illustrating how these practices promote a sense of well-being. Their presentation is a powerful testament to the veracity of this information, as it puts Black voices at the forefront of the narrative about yoga. There is no outside gaze; instead, it is written from the perspective of those with direct knowledge and lived experiences of the Black community. While yoga can be communal, it also holds the power for deeply personal self-reflection. As codified by Patanjali, yoga's very definition helps us see ourselves more clearly.

When I made the decision to transition from yoga practitioner to yoga teacher, I realized the importance of establishing cultural and social roots that would deeply connect me to the practice. It was during my journey to Ghana, West Africa, in search of myself in yoga that I witnessed yoga's presence in daily life, unfolding in a more natural environment. I was awestruck. *Yoga in the Black Community: Healing Practices and Principles* has helped clarify that what I believed was missing in life, much like the hero in Paulo Coelho's *The Alchemist* was always within me. Muhammad and Peppers-Citizen eloquently discuss how yoga aids in the recovery and renewal of our damaged sense of identity. Clues, no matter how small, are always present, waiting to unlock the path to our authentic selves. Our grandparents' stories, the foods our mothers cook, handed down over generations, the knowledge of the vital roles plants and animals play in our lives, and the sparks of creativity within us continuously give birth to transformative gifts such as music, dance, arts, crafts, and fashion, enriching the global community.

Throughout history, across centuries and generations, numerous individuals have emerged as griots, pathfinders, messengers, wisdom keepers, and acharyas, imparting their wisdom to humanity. Even in our present time, these remarkable individuals continue to exist among us, not as celebrities, but as teachers who wholeheartedly aid us in our pursuit of personal transformation.

Yoga offers a process to experience the fullness of our whole being. From colonial times to the present, numerous voices, both past and present, have shaped and informed the African existence in the United States. *Yoga in the Black Community: Healing Practices and Principles* explains how the practical application of yoga today can strengthen our communities, fortify our resilience, and build inner strength. It is a must-read for Black yoga teachers, practitioners, integrative healers, and all those who seek personal growth and expanded knowledge through the practice of yoga.

Foreword

KRISHNA KAUR

I love the straightforward aspects of this book. The concepts are easy to access, as the authors share that the wisdom of yoga can be geared to all; especially to the spirit of Black people at a time when—more than ever—it is deeply needed.

Embracing a yoga lifestyle is invaluable. As one of the early practitioners of yoga in the Black community back in the 1970s, I was personally introduced to kundalini yoga a year and a half after its initial appearance in the United States. I was not planning to walk away from a successful career in the theater, but I had a deep, deep thirst to understand my way to worship God. Kundalini yoga, as taught by Yogi Bhajan, was clear. *If you can't see God in all, you can't see God at all.* Yoga ushered me through the experience of me finding *Me* based on my dedication to the simple yet powerful yoga exercises (kriyas) and simple yet powerful meditations, that continued to wake me up.

When it stops making sense, I said to folks I loved back in the seventies and eighties, *I'm leaving.*

Four decades later, I'm still on my mat sharing the value of yoga in the Black community and beyond.

Acknowledgments

First giving honor to the Creator and Sustainer of the heavens and earth and in the spirit of the West African Akan proverb: *Wuforo dua pa a na ye pia wo* ("He who climbs a good tree is encouraged and supported"), we are honored to acknowledge and thank the communal village who came together to support this project.

Humble bow of gratitude to our families and friends for the encouragement to press forward in completing this project. We nurtured our work for four years before revealing it to our community. When we did, the response of support was overwhelmingly positive. We thank you for giving us the space and time to research, contemplate, and write.

Thanks to our yoga "models"—all budding student practitioners of yoga—for gracing our pages. Thank you for sharing the beautiful expressions of your practice: Tracey Bailey, Jesse Citizen, Oneida Diaz, Nesa Herring, Jeffery Jones, Taj Hakim Martinez, Hadi Muhammad, Iqrama Muhammad, and Sheila Rohan.

Much appreciation to Kathy Donnelly, owner of The Yoga Center of Columbia, Maryland, for graciously opening her yoga center for the photo shoot and beyond.

Thanks to our amazing photographer, Lorenzo Wilkins of SD33 Art Direction & Design, and his assistant, Welton B. Doby, III, assistant photographer. Thank you for your professional eye and patience.

Thanks to our budding photographer, Taj Hakim Martinez, for enriching the mudra section with photos.

Thanks to Judy Omphroy of Move for Fitness, Middletown, Connecticut, for supporting the research on aligning the Christian principles in Part III.

PART I

RESILIENCY IN THE BLACK COMMUNITY

Blacks in America have not forgotten to embrace the connection with this mother of all mothers, earth. Being strangers in a strange land, this connection to nature anchored our resilience to survive.

Introduction:
From Whence We Came

As we arise into the second decade of the 21st century with all of its complexities, it is good to bask in the old school mindset that knows and continues to explore the vast richness of the Black experience in the Western hemisphere. Like the prose of the acapella singing group Sweet Honey in the Rock's spiritual *We Are*, the innate spirit of African American survival is predicated on seeking to know and understand our true nature.

The nature of Black people is indigenous, intrinsic as the elements that sustain the planet earth and our universe. The origin of "home" for Black people is on the continent called Africa, considered to be the cradle of civilization. Indeed, as the birthplace of all life on earth, so the discovery of Lucy,[1] the oldest human remains uncovered in Hadar, Ethiopia, attest, the true nature of human beings is embedded in the foundations of Africa.

This quest to know who we are and where we originated is passed down through six generations of our sojourn in America. In spite of the current politically charged discourse on "critical race theory" (CRT) aimed at lessening the impact of enslavement on Black Americans by some who strive to deny us of the truth of our traumatized history, those of us with this lived experience thirst to know the truth of who we are. Contrary to the distortion of CRT, its inception by leading scholars such as Dr. Kimberlé Williams Crenshaw is the study of the historical impact of racial injustices in America. The intersectionality of systematic racism, sexism, and classism compounds the confusion Black folk experience on a regular basis as we strive to get ahead in a society that professes equal opportunity for all. Often this seeking to understand our life experiences and purpose is what draws us onto the uncommon path of yoga. An uncommon path for many Black Americans, who may misunderstand the practice. Yoga is not a religious observance per se but is often equated with Hinduism that for many Blacks is contrary to their deep Christian familial beliefs.

"The Yoga Sutras [spiritual text] are also commonly known as Raja Yoga, the Royal Yoga," explains the Reverend Jaganath Carrera in his translation of the spiritual text, *Inside the Yoga Sutras*. "They earned this noble status because they present spirituality as a holistic science, universally applicable to people of all faith traditions."[2] For many Black Americans that do practice yoga, do understand it is a universal spirit-led lifestyle that aligns with the fundamental human principles expounded by many faith traditions: freedom, justice, and equality.

This thirst for self-knowledge or "seeking" truth is a natural response for indigenous people. Indigenous African cultures like the Dagara of Ghana, the Igbo of Nigeria, and other peoples of West Africa from Senegal, Benin, Guinea, Sierra Leone, the Ivory Coast, and Cameroon, to name a few of our peoples subjected to enslavement, delight in a tradition of honoring nature as a path to know the source of life. "Our most ancient African ancestors had only themselves, nature and the ability to sense and intuit their life forces and the forces in nature that impacted on their life force," writes the late Dr. John T. Chissell, a physician and founder of the Positive Perceptions Group, an optimal health education network in Baltimore, Maryland. "Nature taught them that in order to survive and thrive, they must be acutely aware of what existed in nature."[3]

The path of yoga, like the indigenous paths of African ancestry, is one of discovering the true Self. The "Self" meaning the ultimate source of life or the Divine. In many Western adaptations of yoga, the 2nd-century South Asian sage Patanjali's ashtanga eight limbs of yoga forms the basis of such practices. Patanjali's eight limbs of yoga, as expressed in his writings, the Yoga Sutras, consist of: yama, right actions toward others; niyama, right actions toward oneself; asana, physical movements through proper alignment of the body, mind, and breath; pranayama, seeking our connection to the life force or prana; pratyahara, withdrawing from relying on what we perceive as the true self; dharana, stilling the mind with focused concentration; dhyana, practicing meditation; and samadhi, experiencing the bliss of knowing the true Self. The eight limbs of yoga are principles and practices for the human journey of life toward the Self. Reminiscent of our quest as Blacks in America to know our true identity, the yogic limb niyama, or personal observances, includes a practice of *ishvara pranidhana*: surrender to the Divine, seeking one's true nature. In Pada 2.45 of the Yoga Sutras, Patanjali explains this practice as *Samadi siddhih ishvarapranidhana*, meaning "from an attitude of letting go into one's source (*ishvara pranidhana*), the state of perfect bliss (*samadhi*) is attained."[4]

The transatlantic slave trade covered 300 years of Europeans extraditing and exporting Blacks from Africa to the Americas from the 16th to 19th centuries. This period of history may be described as the most traumatic experience of a human species' lifetime. Rare is the experience of a people forcibly removed from their homeland, kidnaped, tortured, murdered, and devalued, for the expressed purpose of building a better life for another race of people in spite of themselves. Variations of this experience have impacted Black, Brown, and indigenous people around the globe historically and continue today. However, the history of Africans in America is a tragic one, with generational devastation that continues to erode the Black community as a whole.

Consider national public health research findings such as the Adverse Childhood Experiences (ACE) study directed by the United States Centers for Disease Control (CDC) and Kaiser Permanente. The original ACE study, conducted over a two-year period from 1995 to 1997, explored the impact of exposure to trauma, violence, and neglect during childhood (birth to 17 years of age) on the development of risk factors for chronic health conditions, other diseases, and overall well-being in adults over time.[5] Although this research study was not solely focused on African Americans, each adverse experience codified by the ACE study— for example, chronic physical and mental illness, community violence and aggression, unemployment, drugs and alcohol exposure, limited education, food insecurity, social and environmental turmoil—forms the basis for the majority of African Americans' social determinants of health. Blacks in America have lived with many such adverse experiences since our time of enslavement.

"For most of our country's history," notes professor and behavioral health expert Resmaa Menakem,

> the Black body was forced to serve white bodies. It was seen as a tool, to be purchased from slave traders; stacked on shelves in the bellies of slave ships; purchased at auction; made to plant, weed, and harvest

crops; pressed into service in support of white families' comfort; and used to build a massive agricultural economy. This arrangement was systematically maintained through murder, rape and mutilation, and other forms of trauma, as well as through institutions, laws, regulations, norms, and beliefs.[6]

The American history of slavery demoralized a race of people from many tribes and cultures. Without access to the moral compass that predicated African enslaved people's culture, language, and spiritual faith, our well-being as a community was severely compromised.

While Blacks in America have been removed from their connection to their African homeland and denied access to the knowledge of their self-worth, stepping back to the old school mindset, Blacks in America have not forgotten to embrace the connection with this mother of all mothers—earth. Being strangers in a strange land, this connection to nature anchored our resilience to survive.

Many stereotypes have depicted Africans as savages running nude through jungles with bones in their noses and spears in their hands. Raoul Peck's 2021 documentary, *Exterminate All the Brutes*, highlights the use of these stereotypes as justification for our enslavement. The European creed of Manifest Destiny anchored their belief in a perceived divinely given doctrine that validated their expansion into the Western hemisphere and subjugation of indigenous people. Europeans proclaimed that Black and Brown people were intellectually, morally, and spiritually inferior and thus legitimized their treatment of indigenous people as their superior savior. Nevertheless, from this ancient land and cradle of civilization, we learn the science of plants, medicine, midwifery, architecture, agriculture, music, art, and communication. Gaining access to this knowledge formed the key reason Africans were enslaved to support the building of the Western world and the source of its survival.

Unlike the European capturers, our African ancestors understood their responsibility to the natural world. Their role is stewardship—caretakers that nurtured the earth for future generations. Serving as khalifah or vicegerent (stewards of the earth), humans could and would evolve as long as the earth from whence they came thrived. "Our ancestors had vast medical knowledge and spiritual strength that gave us the resilience to survive our predicament in slavery and colonization."[7]

— CHAPTER 1 —

The Art of Healing

The art of healing to Blacks in America is as innate in our culture as breath is to life. In the face of any critical point in time of crisis, Blacks in America default back into the very nature of ourselves and call on that inner guidance that connects us to the Great Spirit of Creation that we all intuitively know subtly well.

The construct of "healing" has become a hot topic in social media and beyond. Everywhere one looks there are links, discussions, and advertisements about "healing." From Oprah's embrace of WW (formerly known as Weight Watchers) and its claim as the one-stop-shop for wellness, to Dr. Google's 30-second medical advice, everyone it seems has something to say about healing, including contemporary yoga spaces.

Yet what is healing? By formal definition, the meaning of healing is broad and complex. The American Heritage Dictionary defines healing as a process "to restore to health or soundness. To set aright, mend. To restore to spiritual wholeness. To return to health."[1]

In Western study of psychology, healing involves "reordering a person's sense of purpose in the universe," or "the process of evolving one's personality towards greater and more complex wholeness."[2] Healing has also been defined as "the process of bringing together aspects of oneself, body–mind–spirit, at deeper levels of inner knowing, leading towards integration and balance with each aspect having equal importance and value."[3]

The origins of the healing construct are rooted in the Old English lexicon, "hal" meaning "holy; spiritually pure."[4] In the view of the yogic paradigm in which the efficacy of life is in our own hands, we may consider that healing is a birthright, not a privilege for 1% of human beings.

The Yoga Sutras teach us that "By the practice of the limbs of Yoga, the impurities dwindle away and there dawns the light of wisdom leading to discriminative discernment."[5] The Sutra 2.28 reference to the dedication of our lifestyles to the eight limbs of yoga assists us in healing individually and as community, for the commitment to healing oneself cultivates the strong force of love needed to sustain community. The origins of building and sustaining a cohesive Black community in America rely on similar principles to the eight limbs of yoga such as described in a Southern Sotho proverb of South Africa, *Motho ke motho ka batho*, "a person is a person because of other people."[6]

The art of healing to Blacks in America is as essential in our culture as breath is to life. In the face of any critical point in time or crisis, Blacks in America default back into the very nature of ourselves and call on that inner guidance that connects us to the Great Spirit of Creation that we all intuitively know subtly well.

Back in the day, our commitment to community was shaped by external forces of segregation. Often separated from the mainstream of American society, Black communities associated much like the yoga adaptation of the Buddhist concept of sangha: a community of people who share the same values and offer a source of support to all members within the community. In some Buddhist practices "the essence of sangha is awareness, understanding, acceptance, harmony and love."[7]

In segregated communities, enslaved Africans from various tribal cultures learned the value of cooperation as the basis of their survival. Cultural differences that may have caused strife in their homeland were congealed in the melting pot and acceptance of a new "African American" people. "Though they came empty-handed," write curators Mary Elliott and Jazmine Hughes for the *New York Times Magazine*'s 1619 Project, "[enslaved Black people] carried with them memories of loved ones and communities, moral values, intellectual insight, artistic talents and cultural practices, religious beliefs, and skills. In their new environment, they relied on these memories to create new practices and infuse with old ones."[8]

New "sanghas" were harmonized in enslaved Black communities that provided education, apprenticeship, and eldership to secure their livelihood. These sanghas or communities adapted their indigenous spiritual and moral practices along with Christian doctrine to maintain a sense of familial community that was safe and orderly.

From the beginning of their time in the diaspora, Blacks in America depended on each other to ensure the health of their people. Early communities within Black American society included folks who practiced the art of "tuning in" to a spirit greater than self for the healing guidance needed to support the community. Folk healers, farmers, spiritual priests and priestesses, granny midwives, and herbalists kept their fingers on the pulse for seasonal changes of nature, the impact of the contrary ways of American and world societies on the community they lived and served in, and listened (tuned in) to nature's bountiful blessings of healing needed to gird up their people.

The materia medica of Black American healing modalities included embracing the magical and energetic forces within herbs, plants, food, songs, music, prayers, meditation, and always movement. "In the African American epistemology," writes Stephanie Y. Mitchem in *African American Folk Healing*, "the supernatural is not automatically to be feared but to be respected. ... Belief in this power indicates some dimensions of the basic definition of African American folk healing: that human life is understood relationally; it is part of the interconnected shared web of the universe; human life and death are contiguous realms connected by Spirit..."[9]

Various practices of yoga such as kirtan (chanting/singing), pranayama (breath practice), asana (movement), dhyana (meditation)—much like the spiritual practices of praise, song and dance, and ancestral rituals of our African tribal cultural heritage—inform us of our inner connectedness with nature and the ultimate source of our healing. In this, the African American innate connection with Spirit presents a basis for exploring the yoga journey. By way of yoga, the journey is described as the quest to know the true Self. "The transformation of one species into another is brought about by the inflow of nature,"[10] teaches Patanjali in the Kaivalya Pada (chapter) of the Yoga Sutras. Pada 4.2 demonstrates that the transformation we seek may only be achieved by surrendering to that which is the source of our life. The resilience of Blacks in America evolved through our reliance on a faith that our lives and our people matter. This informs our transformational story.

Enslavement is contrary to human nature. It is a practice of control and dominance that will never be won as nature is not designed to be conquered. If humankind were to conquer nature, the world as we know it would cease to exist. This has been proven throughout human history. Societies such as the Greek, Roman, Aztec, and Egyptian empires that grasped for dominance ultimately met their demise. And yet, like the earth, our indigenous nature continues.

— CHAPTER 2 —

Return to Nature

African American spirituality is one of deference to our Creator and praise of gratitude and thanks for their sojourn on earth regardless of their circumstance.

Traditional African healing practices were handed down through our sojourn in America and are some of the jewels that keep our African American culture rich. This chapter explores the most common practices within the vast majority of enslaved Africans that continue to live on in Black American communities today: prayer and praise; herbal medicine; dance; and spirit worship.

Prayer and praise

The act of praying is one of the oldest human practices of communicating with the Divine. Formal and informal acts of supplication and petitioning to gain insight and favor from a higher power center popular modern-day faith tradition from the monotheistic religions (i.e., Judaism, Christianity, and Islam) to the polytheistic faiths (i.e., Hinduism, Buddhism, and Confucianism.)

Various practices of yoga in the West include a ritual of kirtan or chanting. Kirtan is bhakti or praise that is enjoined as a call and response chant, with the lead chanter or singer making the initial call followed by a group response. Just as the religious or spiritual acts of prayer and praise enjoined enslaved Africans to connect with each other and their Creator as they toiled in their fields of labor, the ultimate goal of performing the kirtan is seeking oneness with the Divine.[1]

Indigenous African tribal belief systems also include forms of prayer. Depending on the tribe or region of Africa that Blacks were enslaved from, a wide range of religious or spiritual beliefs were practiced. Blacks in West Africa and the Congo regions (the source of human cargo for enslavement in America) practiced Islam, forms of Judaism, and many tribal polytheistic beliefs including the worship of nature, ancestors, and other deities as the source of the Divine.

Enslaved Blacks in America were often coerced to accept Christianity and were punished for practicing the indigenous beliefs of their native homeland of Africa. "African American religion encompassed non-institutional expressions and activities," reflects Stephanie Y. Mitchem. "Historically in all United States colonies, Africans were forbidden under European religious beliefs from practicing their spiritual beliefs."[2] Most likely, European settlers did not understand the languages of their enslaved captees nor the energetics of their fervor to commune with their God and ancestors to grasp their plight in the diaspora, therefore felt threatened by these unusual acts of devotion. Forcing Christian doctrine on the enslaved provided another avenue of control. Defining or interpreting who is "God" and how best to relate to such a god provided additional insurance for keeping the enslaved Africans in line.

However, enslaved Blacks in America found creative ways of adapting Christian doctrines within their indigenous folk ways, the evolution of praise songs, spirituals, being a key source of resilience during enslavement. Spirituals grew out of a strong desire for freedom and liberation. Enslaved Africans' introduction to the Christian interpretation of the scriptures of the Holy Bible created a kindred relationship with the prophetic and historical accounts of individuals and tribes of people subjected to human atrocities of bondage and affliction reminiscent of their experiences in America. "The nonliterate slaves told the biblical stories by turning them into songs, which when stitched together, recount the Scriptures from beginning to end—from Adam in the garden to John the revelator."[3]

Enslaved Blacks interpreted various prophecies of the Holy Bible as clues to their own freedom and salvation and created spirit-filled songs to inspire each other as they carried the burden of enslaved life. The history of the prophet Moses and his quest to free his people was center stage to enslaved Blacks finding clues to their salvation within the Holy Bible. The spiritual *Go Down Moses* which highlights the historical account of the Old Testament prophet Moses' command to Pharaoh to "let my people go" (Exodus 9:13) was a controversial praise song during enslavement as many slave owners believed it was a call for their enslaved Africans to orchestrate their escape. Yet, the popularity of this spiritual remained strong and was recorded in history by 20th-century music artists such as Louis Armstrong and Paul Robeson.

The Black American civil rights leader, Martin Luther King, Jr.'s famous address at the 1963 March on Washington, *I Have a Dream*, includes lyrics from the slave-based spiritual hymnal *Free at Last*, which depicts the sojourn of enslaved Africans' daily burden and thus reliance on God. Dr. King's inclusion of this passage continued the enslaved Africans' legacy to stand for resilience in the face of adversity.

A fundamental difference in the spiritual practices of enslaved Africans and European Americans was the Christian doctrine of accessing God through Jesus the Christ, and traditional African spiritual practices of communing with God mediated through the intercessions of the ancestors.[4] Ancestors are believed to be closer to the Creator (God), and one's kin could speak to or petition God through one's ancestral line. Reverence for ancestors continues today; in many African American communities the pouring of libations (offering of a liquid or grain) in honor of the ancestors is included in social justice rallies (for example, Black Lives Matter) and in cultural ceremonies such as the First Fruits harvest celebration of Kwanzaa, the Emancipation Day of the enslaved Africans in the southwest, Juneteenth, and during marriages, births, rites of passage, and funerals or home going celebrations.

African American spirituality is one of deference to their Creator and praise of gratitude and thanks for their sojourn on earth regardless of their circumstance. The reliance on our faith punctuated our prayers often through music and song. Negro spirituals evolved through this blending of enslaved Black cultural beliefs, rhythms, and understanding of Christian scriptures. These informal melodies were carried down through oral tradition and some, like *Free at Last*, were later codified under the formal gospel music genre. Further in the diaspora, the roots of reggae music of the Caribbean blend African folklore with Christian based Biblical stories. Lyrics by contemporary reggae musicians, such as Steel Pulse's *Chant a Psalm* and Bob Marley's *Exodus*, intone Biblical scripture as the lived African experience in the Western hemisphere and encourage reliance on our faith as the key to liberation.

Prayer and praise in the Black community is melodic and lyrical. It is the rhythm of the drumbeat that represents the heartbeat of life. Often, like kirtan, these songs of praise are offered as call and response. For the enslaved African and as practiced today in Black churches and during social justice rallies, the call and response is invoked to enjoin a sense of community and oneness.

Prayer and praise in African American spiritual practices displays our emotional connection to the Creator under many names or attributes: God, Christ, Allah, or Jehovah, and is the critical element in our faith and the number one source we seek for healing.

Currently, there are several public health related published studies on the use of complementary and alternative medicine (CAM) by African Americans experiencing various forms of chronic pain. Examples of general CAM modalities include prayer, yoga, meditation, acupuncture, and herbal medicine. The number one CAM modality used by African Americans regardless of age, ailment, or geographic location (rural or urban) is prayer.

For example, a study of African American adolescents living in urban areas noted 61% of participants reporting prayer as the CAM modality most often used and efficacious in relieving asthma related symptoms.[5] An integrative review of research publications on the use of CAM by African American cancer survivors highlights the use of prayer as the primary tool employed to support emotional and mental well-being.[6]

The essence of African American self-care is our foundational belief in a higher power. The ideal of our innate ability to heal ourselves is our belief in the possibility of a power greater than our own.

"Home remedies," herbal medicine

Reliance on the use of plants as medicine became a staple for enslaved Africans' health. Understandably, due to a chasm of distrust of the Europeans who enslaved them to an environment that often resulted in their death and disease, African Americans preferred to rely on the faith healing methods rooted in their own beliefs and cultures.

The application of plants as medicine is as old as mankind. Historical recordings of the use of plant medicine are noted in the hieroglyphs found in the pyramids in Egypt, Mexico, and South America and in both religious historical records noted in Biblical and Islamic scriptures. Many such plants mentioned in both the Old and New Testaments of the Holy Bible as well as in the Holy Qur'an are common culinary spices used today, such as garlic, sage, and flaxseed, and are known from contemporary research studies as plants with healing properties for supporting our physical organ systems.[7] Enslaved Africans used both garlic (*Allium sativum*) and sage (*Salvia officinalis*) as poultices and teas for illness.[8] Similar to the contemporary research on the use of flaxseed (*Linum usitatissimum*) enslaved Africans were known to brew flax tea to ease digestive upset.[9]

The science of plant medicine has been codified in indigenous medical sciences such as the Arabic medicine classified by Avicenna (Ibn Sina) in the *Canon of Medicine* and the medical practice of ayurveda in India. These historical medical sciences as well as other traditional practices by aboriginal peoples around the world considered plants as life-giving sources of vitality. In India for example, the "coordinated or integrated usage of herbs was based upon the ancient Ayurvedic science of herbal energetics. In this is a system for determining the qualities and powers of herbs according to the laws of nature, so that herbs can be used objectively and specifically according to individual conditions."[10]

Nature provides sustenance within all of its elements that both nourishes and cures all life forms. Plant medicine is relational to humans and animals alike based on geographic location. As humans and animals adapt to the climates that they live in, native species of plants in those areas provide us with a source of food and medicine.

For enslaved Africans, adaptation to America and their survival was grounded on the ability to understand this foreign environment. To gain mastery of their surroundings, enslaved Blacks may possibly have imported a practice similar to the "Doctrine of Signatures": the discovery of a plant's medicinal qualities by observing the signs (signatures) left by God.[11] For example, the shape of a plant's leaves or flowering part may indicate its healing properties, such as eyebright (*Euphrasia rostkoviana*), its flowering bud resembling an eye therefore it may be applied for certain eye conditions. Vegetation, too, follows this doctrine: tomatoes resembling the shape of the heart with medicinal properties of vitamin C and quercetin provide beneficial antioxidant molecules to support cardiovascular health. The walnut resembles the human brain, and its rich source of essential fatty acids provides an abundance of nutrients for brain development.

Comparably, foundational to ayurveda, the sister science of yoga, is the belief that every individual is a unique expression of the creation and is a microcosm of the universe. "As above so below, as below so above": the study of nature and the universe gives us "signs" from the Divine to understand our true dosha or nature. Ayurveda, like other traditional indigenous healing sciences such as traditional Chinese medicine (TCM), employs the healing properties of plants as foundational to medicine.

Reliance on the use of plants as medicine became a staple for enslaved Africans' health. Understandably, due to a chasm of distrust of the Europeans who enslaved them to an environment that often resulted in their death and disease, African Americans preferred to rely on the faith healing methods rooted in their own beliefs and cultures. "During centuries of oppression and poverty, African Americans were often isolated from even rudimentary medical care and therefore developed their own healing traditions using easily accessible herbs, foodstuffs, and other substances."[12]

Over time, a pharmacopeia of home remedies was employed in African American communities around the country and handed down through generations. The use of pot licker consisting of a broth of boiled brassica vegetables (e.g., collard greens, kale, cabbage) was known by enslaved Africans in the southern regional states of America to support common colds and tummy upsets. Black folks in the north employed a mustard plaster: a poultice of mustard seeds, cayenne pepper, and eucalyptus wrapped in a damp cloth for lung infections like bronchitis. An infusion of eyebright tea was cooled and applied as an eye wash for sties. The bright yellow flowers and green leaves of mullein (*Verbascum thapsus*) supported all forms of congestion in the upper respiratory tract. This belief in the power of plants was based on enslaved Africans, relationships and trust of the elders in the community.

Today, this knowledge continues to be grounded with our elders for future generations of young Black Americans seeking to know and apply ancient healing wisdom. Consider the works of Lucretia VanDyke, herbalist and author of the book *African American Herbalism: A Practical Guide to Healing Plants and Folk Traditions*. VanDyke's work is a contemporary exploration of the use of indigenous plant medicine practices to promote health and well-being in the Black community.

Millennial Indy Srinath is carrying the tradition of plant medicine as an urban farmer and social media influencer. Srinath shares her knowledge of plants with younger generations through hands-on gardening demonstrations and most recently, in her televised series for National Geographic, *Farming is Life*.

Organizations such as WANDA (Women Advancing Nutrition, Dietetics, and Agriculture) are supporting the legacy of cultural healing as a Black woman-led social justice movement. Carrying the legacy of

African knowledge of plants and food as medicine, WANDA's aim is to "educate, advocate and innovate to achieve nutrition equity" for the Black community and beyond.[13]

Dance as a spiritual practice

For Africans in America, the drumbeat of our culture is steeped in movement. Music, song, and praying were seldom experienced without the physical presence of swaying or dancing. The joy of movement created a whole body (holistic) experience to healing: the mind, body, and spirit moving as one toward better well-being.

Observing the hatha yoga vinyasa practice *surya namaskar* (sun salutation) as it flows through 12 continuous asana or postures, one sees the resemblance of the Salat prayer service of the Islamic faith. In fact, the value of movement in spiritual practices is being validated as vital to our physical health and well-being.

Dr. Stephen Porges' work on polyvagal theory explores the physiology of human emotions through the autonomic nervous system. Porges theorizes that the polyvagal system is grounded in the ancient healing arts and that mindful practices like yoga and meditation and spiritual practices such as the Islamic prayer service support our physical health and mental well-being.[14]

In the research paper "The Islamic prayer (Salah/Namaaz) and yoga togetherness in mental health," which compares the benefits of the Islamic prayer service with the practice of yoga, the authors note that "a closer look at these two forms of worship reveal a number of similarities in their physical execution and the accrued medical and psychological improvements in the life quality of the practitioner."[15]

Liturgical or praise dance in African American churches is also reminiscent of the sun salutation vinyasa as the movements of these dances are expressions of the spirit of the Divine flowing through the body of the dancer. Often liturgical expressions led the dancer to points similar to the yogic practice principle of samadhi (ecstasy), such dancers experiencing being "slain in the spirit" or touched by God.

Dancing—moving rhythmically in tune with the energetic forces of nature offered through the base drumbeat of music—is one of the oldest expressions of love for the Divine in indigenous cultures. In Indigenous peoples of America's cultures, much like African indigenous cultures, the steady drumbeat ushered in the call to the Creator with practitioners dancing, chanting, and praying.

For Africans in America, the drumbeat of our culture is steeped in movement. Music, song, and praying were seldom experienced without the physical presence of swaying or dancing. The joy of movement created a whole body (holistic) experience to healing: the mind, body, and spirit moving as one toward better well-being. The healing benefits of dancing include strengthening the cardiovascular and immune systems and enhancing mood.[16]

Dance has always been important to African Americans as a principal means of self-expression.[17] African Americans dance in their homes, outdoors during play, at all family celebrations including weddings, births, and funerals. During enslavement and in contemporary times, dancing provided Blacks with a means of finding and expressing joy that tapped into the source of resilience needed to sustain them through the traumas of life. One of the earliest forms of Black dance acknowledged during enslavement is the "ring shout." The ring shout follows choreographical movements that enslaved Africans performed as a spiritual experience to bless their lives as they moved about their daily strifes from labor to love.

Throughout our history, dancing in African American culture took on many forms and is performed for pleasure as well as in rituals. Dancer, choreographer, and anthropologist Katherine Dunham devoted her life work to the study of the culture of dance as a spiritual medium for Africans living in the diaspora. "There is something in the dance of religious ecstasy that has always made me feel that through this exercise man might come into his own, be freed of inferiority and guilt in the face of whatever might be his divinity," Dunham writes in her second autobiography *Island Possessed*.[18]

The value of African dance and praise for maintaining the history and health of African American culture influences many forms of movement today from hip hop, ballet, and contemporary modern to popular line and hand dancing. The choreography of Black performing artists such as the late Geoffrey Holder and his wife and artistic partner Carmen de Lavallade – Holder himself, a practitioner of Theosophy – credits this spiritual study and meditation to grounding his creative work. Within these spiritual practices, Holder was able to focus on the various artistic crafts that came naturally to him and thus he was successful in many artistic venues such as visual arts, dance, choreography, and as an actor, director, and producer.

Holder's choreography often blended indigenous traditions. For a signature work created for the Dance Theatre of Harlem, Holder entitled the ballet *Dougla*, explaining, "Where twain meet, Hindu and African tangle, their offspring are called Dougla."[19]

Most notably, the works by the Alvin Ailey American Dance Theater solidified the soul of our sojourn in America through ballet creations that were based on Ailey's "blood memories."[20] Ailey strived to create dance that honors and reflects Black culture. His storytelling through choreography voices the history of the Black American experience and especially African American expression of spiritual worship as depicted in the Black ballet saga *Revelations*. Based on Negro spirituals including *Fix Me Jesus*, *Sinner Man*, *Wade in the Water*, *Rock My Soul*, and *Lazarus*, *Revelations* tells the story of African American resilience through their faith in the Divine. Ailey believed that our Black history is stored in our bodies and that through dance we bring these stories alive.

Visionary dancer, choreographer, and social justice activist Jawole Willa Jo Zollar founded Urban Bush Women, a "performance ensemble dedicated to exploring the use of cultural expression as a catalyst for social change."[21] Zollar's work is recognized as foundational to the continuing legacy of African dance in the diaspora as a means of assisting American culture to make sense of the traumatic aspects of enslaved Africans' experiences and empowering the Black community to take action through the arts and beyond.

The late Chuck Davis, founding director of Dance Africa, developed this annual festival of performing arts dedicated to African dance and traditions celebrated through the lens of African American culture. In addition, performing arts companies such as the Bill T. Jones/Arnie Zane Dance Company continue the legacy of African dance in America that inspires young Black dancers and choreographers to "embody our choices in using our voices."[22]

Spirit worship

Healing is central to indigenous African spirituality. Healing the relationships between people, between people and the spirit world, and between people and their ancestors is key to maintaining a healthy community.

African American spirit worship is magical. It comes in a variety of forms that explores the mysteries of the supernatural in order to understand the innate edicts of nature and make sense of the world that we live in. Such spiritual practices were born during enslavement and are adaptations of spiritual veneration practices from the homeland of Northern West Central Africa. As noted earlier, enslaved Africans were forbidden from practicing any other religion aside from the Christian religion adopted by European settlers.

The heart of enslaved African spirituality is communing with the Divine essence of nature. This spirituality is based on the indigenous Africans' embrace of a universal concept of "being" where mind, body, and spirit are one and cannot be separated. Enslaved Africans believed that all elements of nature—including plants, trees, rocks, earth, waters, and animals—hold divine energy and interact with human life. The belief that the ancestors, angels, and other deities of the supernatural intercede on their behalf is systematized in various practices such as vodun and hoodoo. Two of the most misunderstood and misrepresented spiritual practices in the West, each has an established set of disciplines that support the well-being of human beings through the practitioner's ability to tap into the cosmic energy of the Divine.

Closely related to the yogic concept of karma, an aspect of customs found in vodun and hoodoo supports the perception that a person's interest is influenced by their own actions, the reactions of others, and one's past actions in other lifetimes. A person's deeds may gain the admiration of other spirits (deities) or the ancestors or admonishment by the same. In such cases, various remedies—plants and herbs, chanting, and conjure (summoning into existence an action or thing by magic)—may be applied to remedy such situations. Healing is central to indigenous African spirituality. Healing the relationships between people, between people and the spirit world, and between people and their ancestors is key to maintaining a healthy community.

Hoodoo and vodun are often used interchangeably; however, depending on the region of the United States, the practices differ significantly. Vodun or "spirit" in the Fon, Gun, and Ewe languages of West Africa is considered a religious practice. It is "a religion of creation and life. It is the worship of the sun, the water, and other natural forces"[23] and is acculturated throughout the various tribes of northwestern central regions of Africa and thus was transported to the Western hemisphere during the enslavement period.

33

Unlike the monotheistic religions or certain polytheistic faiths, vodun does not include written scriptural text. The practice is based on oral tradition and is preserved through rituals of songs and dance, where the bodies of practitioners are initiated into the faith through various acts of worship. Spiritual leaders (*houngan*/men and *mambos*/ women) guide initiates through rituals of transcendence during which a pantheon of deities or gods (*loa*) influence human life. Through the music, song, and dance, practitioners reach a trance-like state during which *loa* may mount and ride the person spiritually in order to communicate to the vodun *humofor* (community) that called them forth.

During enslavement, vodun was practiced in the southern region of Louisiana and the Gulf as well as in the Caribbean, especially Haiti and Cuba. The 21st century finds vodun practitioners throughout the United States, Caribbean, and South America. In Philadelphia, for example, America's first church of voodoo—Le Peristyle Haitian Sanctuary—traces its roots back to a 500-year-old vodun lineage in Mariani, Haiti.[24] In alignment with enslaved African spiritual journeys in the West, the Le Peristyle Haitian Sanctuary blends voodoo practices within a Christian-like church religion, professing a belief in one God and in the Holy Loa (as the Holy Spirit).[25]

Hoodoo, on the other hand, incorporates rituals that influence human behavior. Hoodoo, or conjure, was primarily practiced in the southeastern Atlantic region (North and South Carolina, Georgia, and Florida) and its origins include African, Indigenous peoples of America, and European spiritual practices and influences. Often considered a source of "black magic," herbal remedies, incantations, prayers, and sacrifices are performed for various purposes such as attracting love or money or repelling bad luck or evil. Much like other forms of spirituality, the aim of hoodoo practices is healing.

Hoodoo's bad reputation was born during the 19th century, primarily in Haiti where the enslaved Africans used the practice as a focal point for their liberation. Many of the Haitian slave uprisings and the ultimate island-wide revolution that led to the first independent Black nation in the Western hemisphere was proclaimed through hoodoo. Subsequently, the hoodoo "black magic" persona was cast by European Americans as something to be feared and therefore attacked and destroyed. This "othering" of hoodoo and other Africana spirituality, according to Yvonne Chireau, professor of religious studies at Swarthmore College, aligns with racist tactics employed to subdue enslaved Africans and their offspring for generations. Professor Chireau's research concluded that the practice of hoodoo is a "healing modality that transcends the boundaries of the self."[26] In contemporary practices of hoodoo, according to Professor Chireau, this healing is necessary to address the afflictions of social inequalities and injustice experienced by Black people. Subsequently, Hoodoo practices are being employed as rituals of protest and resistance in many BIPOC (Black, Indigenous, People of Color) communities around the United States.

Hoodoo practitioners such as Denise Alvarado, a prolific writer on southern folk traditions, have authored books and developed academic courses to preserve hoodoo practice within mainstream society. Alvarado's Crossroads University[27] and American Rootwork Association's (ARA) academic journal are dedicated to researching the science that underlies the "black magic" of hoodoo.

"While much of African Americans' religious heritage was destroyed by the hardship inherent in slavery and by many Blacks' willing conversion to Christianity," writes Jeffrey E. Anderson in *Conjure in African American Society*, "it retained a vital niche in their folk beliefs."[28] Aspects of African spirit worship have been adapted in various contemporary Christian churches with customs such as worshippers "catching the Holy Ghost"; being "slain in the spirit"; and receiving prophecy from the Holy Spirit about current conditions or future events.

— CHAPTER 3 —

The Call and Response

The health disparity and morbidity of living life as Black in 21st century America dictates the urgency needed to reconnect to traditions that sustained our well-being.

The ebb and flow of African American migratory patterns in and out of the countryside and into urban inner cities was due to the economic whims of American society's institutionalized segregation. "Many [Black] folks abandoned...the use of traditional healing during the great migration to the northern states,"[1] seeking promises of opportunity for a better life. Subsequently, the sense of community among Blacks in America has been stifled as the unifying force that holds our culture together, and thus our traditional ways of healing are somewhat lost.

Fortunately, Blacks in America survived by using oral traditions of imparting knowledge. For generations, our traditional healing modalities were passed on in a relay hand-off pattern elder to child in the race against time. In the absence of this sense of community, the Black oral healing tradition has become like a cultural endangered species. And yet, as Stephanie Y. Mitchem writes, "African American folk healing is not a closed system; it is not frozen in time, and it is not limited to a single place. Instead, African American folk healing is adaptable to different conditions and, like any aspect of a living culture, changes."[2]

As the communal Black family scattered throughout the four corners of North America, the spirit of Black American resilience prevailed, and a universal leadership of healers stepped up to keep Black healing traditions known. The African American traditions of healing were held, protected, and passed down through the centuries by Black leadership whose spirits were energized to embrace this sacred knowledge.

The African traditions of healing through diet and herbal medicine were systematized by our spiritual pioneers such as the Honorable Elijah Muhammad (*How to Eat to Live*), Dick Gregory (*Natural Diet for Folks Who Eat: Cookin' with Mother Nature*), Dr. Llaila O. Afrika (*African Holistic Health*), and Alfredo "Dr. Sebi" Bowman (*Nutritional Guide for Healthy Living*). These pioneers challenged the quality of the standard American diet and the enslaved Africans' adaptation of this diet as the leading cause of illness with the Black community.

The Honorable Elijah Muhammad was an early proponent of what is now merchandised as "intermittent fasting," urging his followers and readers to eat "one meal a day."[3] He also understood and taught the value of both physical and spiritual food. "The earth is full of food: but good health cannot enter our bodies until we have the proper food in the body and the proper food for thought," Muhammad writes in *How to Eat to Live, Book One*. "If we do not have the proper food for our way of thinking, we still cannot enjoy peace, good health, joy and gladness of heart."[4]

Dick Gregory's wit charms his readers to transition from the Standard American Diet (SAD) to a vegetarian lifestyle and regain our Afrocentric healing practices such as fasting. "When I speak of religious fasting," Gregory writes, "I mean fasting for the purpose of heightened spiritual awareness. It is an act of piety of freeing oneself from the demands of bodily appetites to be in closer communion with Mother Nature, the Ground of Being, God, the Supreme Being or whatever name one chooses to call the Universal Force and Intelligence."[5]

Dr. Llaila O. Afrika's book includes the use of Africana herbal materia medica to support common diseases and health challenges affecting African Americans. Afrika notes that although Black cultural influences in America are evident in styles of clothing, hairstyles, music, and dance, "one major step has been overlooked in this process: the reclaiming of African herbal medicine and holistic natural food diet and lifestyle."[6]

The late Dr. Sebi influenced the millennial generation to embrace a holistic lifestyle predicated on vegetarian diet, herbal supplements, and the cultivation of self-love and self-confidence. Following the yogic principle of *svadhyaya* (self-study), Sebi's own health challenges led him into the journey of healing. A native of Honduras, Alfredo "Dr. Sebi" Bowman immigrated to the United States while suffering from several chronic diseases that plague the Blacks in the diaspora: asthma, diabetes, and obesity. He used his own health conditions as a means of studying human physiology and the botanical healing aspects of plants. Sebi developed a line of herbal dietary supplements that remains contro-versial to this day. However, hip hop artists such as the late Lisa "Left-Eye" Lopes and Nipsey Hussle, along with celebrities such as Michael Jackson and John Travolta, credit Sebi's holistic treatment strategies of detoxification through fasting, vegetarian diet, and herbal medicine targeted to decrease inflammation and congestion by supporting cellular integrity with restoring their health and well-being.[7]

In 2020 holistic health practitioner Khetnu Neter founded the Gul-lah Geechee Herbal Gathering: A Conference for Black and Indigenous Herbalists and Community. The annual gathering is convened in the sea islands of South Carolina, where the descendants of the Gullah Geechee people of West and Central Africa were enslaved. With Black and indigenous healers from around the United States sharing the ancient wisdoms of their ancestors, the gathering provides opportunities for participants to "converge, educate, heal and uplift each other."[8]

The sacredness of prayer and praise became a universal act of spiri-tuality outside of the institutions of religion. Iyanla Vanzant (*Mastering Peace, Affirmative Prayer for Guidance, Reflection and Healing*) and the healing soulful songs of Dr. Bernice Johnson Reagon's Sweet Honey in the Rock represent two powerful voices that honored the call and response of our ancestors.

The traditional African healing arts have influenced the practice of yoga in the Black community. One such high profile influence was Alice Coltrane, whose artistic vision and music placed her on a spiritual jour-ney that embraced yoga and inspired other musicians and performers to express their spirituality through the arts. Like many African Americans, the significance of Alice Coltrane's spiritual journey began in the church. "Alice Coltrane always remained deeply connected to the African Amer-ican spiritual and musical locus of her family's origins."[9] In 1970 Alice Coltrane met spiritual teacher Swami Satchidananda and dedicated her life to the spiritual path of yoga. Blessed with the Sanskrit name meaning "Transcendental Lord's Highest Song of Bliss," Alice Turiyasangitananda founded the Vedantic Center in Southern California. As Swamini Alice Turiyasangitananda, she dedicated her music in the style of kirtan or praise for the Divine.

Another yoga pioneer, Krishna Kaur, studied kundalini yoga under Yogi Bhanjan who initiated his interpretation of kundalini during the 1960s. Kundalini is a yoga practice that focuses on kriyas. Kriya, as defined in the Yoga Sutras of Patanjali (Pada 2.1), means devotion through the discipline of purification, study, and effort.[10] Kriyas as practiced in Yogi Bhajan's kundalini yoga include asana (body postures), mudras (energetic hand positions), pranayama (breathwork), mantras (intentional, repeated sounds), bandhas (constriction of particular area of the body), drishti (directing the gaze of the eyes), and savasana (relaxation).[11]

Krishna Kaur taught the practice of kundalini and kriyas throughout the United States and Mexico, focusing on inner city communities. She founded Y.O.G.A. for Youth: a non-profit organization dedicated to teaching yoga teachers to work with at-risk youth, in schools and juvenile facilities.[12]

Increasing in popularity with Blacks in America and worldwide is an African-centered form of yoga, kemetic yoga, that follows the philosophy, principles, and practices of ancient Egyptian texts on mind–body–spirit development. "Kemetic yoga is the ancient Egyptian system of yoga enlightenment based upon the practices of physical movements, combined with controlled deep breathing and meditation."[13] Two leaders in this work are Sebai Dr. Muata Ashby and Yirser Ra Hotep.

Dr. Muata Ashby is a historical researcher and founder of the Sema Institute of Yoga, a non-profit organization dedicated to spreading the wisdom of yoga and ancient Egyptian mystical traditions. Muata Ashby authored a collection of works, *Egyptian Yoga: The Philosophy of Enlightenment*, that chronicles the history of yoga as an ancient lifestyle originating in the early civilizations of India and East Africa (Indus, Egypt/Kamit, and Ethiopia/Kush). Muata Ashby's research findings establish Egyptian civilization as the cradle of humanity and a major influence on all mind–body–spirit philosophies. Early civilizations in Asia and Europe "espoused the same philosophy that had existed in Egypt for many thousands of years."[14] Various schools of spiritual thought such as Christianity, Hinduism, Buddhism, and the Kabbalah share similar doctrines of belief for the overall spiritual advancement of man.[15]

Yirser Ra Hotep is the master instructor of kemetic yoga in the United States. He created the Yoga Skills Method, a kemetic style of yoga that practices asana (postures) by creating the forms of Egyptian hieroglyphics. Kemetic yoga is practiced at a slow, methodical pace that emphasizes movement with the breath. During the 1970s Yirser Ra Hotep along with his teacher, master instructor Dr. Asar Ha-pi, developed the original research documenting kemetic yoga. Yirser Ra Hotep continues to teach and train kemetic yoga instructors in the United States and throughout Africa and the African diaspora.

A champion of Black woman goddess power, holistic healing and kemetic yoga practitioner Queen Afua employs ancient African knowledge to inspire millions of people throughout the United States and the world to "heal thyself" with plant-based medicine, yoga, meditation, and energy work. Queen Afua also employed the yogic principle of *svadhyaya* (self-study) as a young teen suffering from chronic health conditions asthma, eczema, premenstrual syndrome (PMS), and headaches. She credits Dick Gregory's *Natural Diet for Folks Who Eat: Cookin' with Mother Nature* as her source for taking up the healing mantle. A self-proclaimed zealot for holistic health, Queen Afua's work urges the Black community to embrace the "African Natural Lifestyle; by imbibing our culture we will never be sick."[16]

Holding the container for the sangha of Black yoga teachers, the Black Yoga Teachers Alliance (BYTA) was founded in 2009 by Dr. Maya Breuer and Jana Long. BYTA is a "collective of yoga teachers who share the peace and power of yoga to inspire conscious living." Its mission is "to support the educational and professional development of black yoga teachers."[17] Jana Long produced the film *The Uncommon Yogi* for BYTA, to chronicle the history of yoga in the African American community.

These and other African American healing arts pioneers continue the legacy of resilience by lecturing, preaching, and teaching various aspects of supporting healthy lifestyles for the Black community.

"Why take an African centered approach to optimal health in this day and age?" writes John T. Chissell:

> Anthropologists, paleontologists, and geneticists (studying mitochondrial DNA) are all confirming through these scientific disciplines that the original human beings are of African descent. As Earth's first human inhabitants, Africans have the longest history of knowing based on life experience, and consequently, laws of living based on life lessons would have had to have started with the ancient Africans and been passed down to us (their survivors) having been tested by time. These laws of living, now known as Universal Laws, Universal Principles, or Natural Laws, when incorporated into our own lives, can do much to eliminate the fear and confusion so prevalent in our current populations due to the way we have all been programmed by much of the media and marketing we are continuously exposed to.[18]

The health disparity and morbidity of living life as Black in 21st-century America dictates the urgency needed to reconnect to traditions that sustained our well-being. Age, financial difficulties, living alone, smoking, pain-related chronic medical conditions, and depressive symptoms are associated with pain intensity in African Americans.[19] And yet, "African Americans use more praying, hoping and emotion-focused coping strategies than Caucasians."[20]

In the 21st century, traditional "folk" healing has a new persona in the form of complementary and alternative medicine (CAM), the Western cultural attempt at codifying indigenous healing modalities in relation to standards of allopathic medicine. Nevertheless, the origins of allopathic medicine are rooted in many of the old ways of healing. The pharmaceutical pharmacopeia, for example, is predicated on herbal plant remedies and often uses synthetic replications of a plant's phytochemical compounds.[21]

In a study on the use of CAM in a local African American community in Philadelphia, African American participants who used CAM "felt that the use of [CAM] remedies...enabled them to be more in control of their health," and "that they felt empowered by their ability to manage their own healthcare."[22]

Yoga as a CAM practice of self-care is expanding its boundaries. Indeed "lifetime yoga practitioners are more likely female, non-Hispanic white and college educated, however Hispanic and non-Hispanic Blacks are increasingly using yoga in the USA." [23]

John T. Chissell reminds us that

> We are here by the grace of the Creator of nature and the universe, and we are meant to be in charge of lives filled with joy, radiant health, and meaningful work, worship, and play. Certain of our wise ancient African ancestors since the beginning of time moved through their lives with growing awareness that when we humans learn, think, and act according to the laws of nature and the universe, we move automatically toward our greatest potential and highest good.[24]

PART II

HEALTH DISPARITIES IN THE BLACK COMMUNITY

Mistrust of healthcare has its roots in enslaved life in the United States. Unethical research practices also contributed to a lack of trust in people and systems that conduct research. Thoughts about perceived discrimination, and beliefs that HIV/AIDS is a racial warfare weapon, a strategy to reduce the Black population by requiring condoms, are but two of the conspiracy theories.[1] And, more recently, COVID-19 had a substantial effect on the Black community.

— CHAPTER 4 —

Health Equity:
A Historical Perspective

The mental and physical health of millions of people is negatively affected by racism, both interpersonal and structural, and it prevents them from attaining their highest level of health...

The desire to live a healthy life, health equity, continues to be a daunting challenge for Black Americans. Health equity, an environment in which everyone has the opportunity to achieve their highest level of health, was defined by organizations such as the National Academies of Sciences, Engineering, and Medicine, the Centers for Disease Control and Prevention (CDC), and the American Public Health Association.[1] In general, health equity is present when everyone has the opportunity to gain full health and no one is disadvantaged because they do not have access to social, economic, environmental, or structural resources.

As early as colonial America, the effect of racism began to influence the health of those who called America home. The American public structure of systemic disparities resulted in Black American health equity vulnerabilities in the areas of income, employment, education, transportation, and access to food and healthcare. These disparities adversely impact the people that face these obstacles.[2]

Racism is a system of structuring opportunity and assigning value based on the social interpretation of how one looks (which is what we call "race"), that unfairly disadvantages some individuals and communities, unfairly advantages other individuals and communities, and saps the strength of the whole society through the waste of human resources.[3]

The 21st-century outlook for the overall health and well-being of Blacks in America paints a daunting picture. Black Americans' trials during their sojourn in the diaspora resulted in morbidity and mortality rates that outpace not only White American society but any and all other races and cultures that migrate to the North American hemisphere in search of a free, just, and equal society.

The American Public Health Association stated that "racism is a system of policies and practices where the color of a person's skin determines their value resulting in them being disadvantaged."[4] Over time, racism in the United States permeated the country's institutional, societal, and mental foundations, and how we experience everyday living, presenting deeply seated roots of racism across generations of Black and non-Black people.[5]

This systemic racism occurs when opportunities and outcomes are built into or are part of how a system operates. The institutional foundations include organizational policies and practices. Societal foundations include both state and federal laws and programs, and culture. How we learn and our memories, attitudes, beliefs, and values are included in our individual mental foundations, while our habits and activities are part of our everyday living.[6]

How Black people are treated in the United States is a public health issue proven to be a basis for health inequities.[7] In 1903 W.E.B. DuBois stated that "the problem of the 20th Century is the problem of the color line." The problem of the color line still exists. People of the global majority still experience racism and the racism impacts their health. The phrase now frequently used is "people of color" or BIPOC, Black, Indigenous, People of Color. But the term people of global majority, PGM, has a richer meaning. It includes people who are Black, indigenous to the global south, Brown, Asian, dual-heritage, and people who have been racialized as ethnic minorities.

Blogger Daniel Lim talks about his views about identification and states that the term "people of color" centers Whiteness even as it attempts to be an affirming identity label for non-White people.[8] It perpetuates the idea that Whiteness is the default and White people therefore have no particular race. Race is a special identity marker that is only assigned to people who are not White; who are the *other*. Race comes with color. Non-White people are subsequently *of color* by virtue of not being color-free, White people. The term "people of color" situates non-White people's existence in strict relation to Whiteness, rather than liberating them from it.

The mental and physical health of millions of people is negatively affected by racism, both interpersonal and structural, and it prevents them from attaining their highest level of health, consequently affecting the health of our nation.[9] It can be deliberate or thoughtless and it operates at different levels within society.

A historical perspective

Dr. James McCune Smith was the first African American to earn a medical degree, in the mid-1800s. He was a leading voice in the profession and argued that health reflected a person's membership in groups created by a race-based society structure. Dr. Smith articulated that health disparities linked America's racial caste system to inequitable social conditions and that racism caused health inequities, leading to health disparities. Dr. Smith's arguments were scientifically validated in the 1899 sociological study of Black Americans by Dr. William Edward Burghardt DuBois (W.E.B. DuBois). The study, *The Philadelphia Negro*, explained that social factors like economics, sanitation, and education led to racial differences in mortality in Philadelphia, not innate racial traits or tendencies. Dr. DuBois reported that white supremacy contributed to structural poverty and higher levels of disease and death. Dr. Smith and Dr. Dubois were pioneers who identified that racism, not race, is the cause of health disparities.[10]

Over the last 50 years scientific racism, the idea that Black people are biologically, intellectually, and morally inferior, has been somewhat less evident in mainstream society due to social movements that have demanded full citizenship for Black Americans. Despite United States civil rights legislation (e.g., Civil Rights Bill of 1866, Civil Rights Act of 1964, Voting Rights Act of 1965, and Civil Rights Act of 1968), that advocated for prohibiting discrimination in public spheres and for civic participation, structural racism, bias, and other forms of harmful discrimination persist today. There are several factors that contribute to continuing health disparities in Black communities.[11]

These factors include implicit and explicit provider biases, mistrust of the medical institutions and medical providers, low self-esteem in individuals, stereotyping, and racism. The 1985 Heckler Report (Report of the Secretary of the United States Department of Health and Human Services Task Force on Black and Minority Health) formalized the first assessment of racial health disparities. According to the Heckler Report there were six leading preventable causes of death (cancer, cardiovascular disease, diabetes, infant mortality, chemical dependency, and homicide/ unintentional injury) in the Black population as compared to the White population.[12] Twenty years later, the Institute of Medicine Report on Unequal Treatment followed with a similar finding that highlighted disparities in healthcare and racism can impact the health outcomes of individuals considered to be part of minority groups. Both reports led to more interest in population health and how racism and social factors affect clinical outcomes.[13]

In the United States race is a major consideration when determining socioeconomic status. Therefore, it should not come as a surprise that racial disparities in socioeconomic status would result from race-based policies related to what some believe to be racial inferiority. Actually, the term "racial inferiority" itself produces racial disparities. The term "structural racism" also describes inequities that appear as racialized access to resources and opportunities that the dominant White society codifies in laws, policies, and even societal norms.[14] It is a term that encapsulates the ways that inequities endure by denying access to the resources, opportunities, and services that laws, policies, practices, and societies say are available to the dominant White society. It is difficult to identify a particular culprit responsible for denying access to marginalized populations and this makes it difficult to identify the perpetrator or bring an end to the disparities. It is easy to deny that the inequities exist.[15]

Several 20th-century works, such as *Caste, Class and Race*, *Black Metropolis*, and *An American Dilemma*, explain how structural racism creates and perpetuates poverty. Communities of racial and ethnic minorities are the result of structurally racist policies and practices. Related factors include unemployment, poor education, and inadequate housing.[16]

Couple the lack of investment in progress in the domains of social determinants in race-based communities with the absence of health programs, and Black, Hispanic, Indigenous peoples of America, and non-English speaking immigrants and refugees are condemned to live in poverty and to be afflicted by substandard health.[17]

CHAPTER 5

Environmental Inequities and Health

Our health is determined in part by access to social and economic opportunities. The conditions in which we live explain in part why some Americans are healthier than others and why Americans more generally are not as healthy as they could be.

Health starts in our homes, schools, workplaces, neighborhoods, and communities. We know that taking care of ourselves, by eating well and staying active, not smoking, getting the recommended immunizations and screening tests, and seeing a doctor when we are sick can influence our health. Our health is also determined in part by access to social and economic opportunities. The conditions in which we live explain in part why some Americans are healthier than others and why Americans more generally are not as healthy as they could be.

The growing body of research shows that centuries of racism in this country profoundly impacts communities of color. The impact is pervasive and deeply embedded in our society. Data show that racial and ethnic minority groups throughout the United States experience higher rates of illness and death across a wide range of health conditions, when compared to their White counterparts. Additionally, the life expectancy of non-Hispanic Black Americans is four years lower than that of White Americans. The COVID-19 pandemic, and its disproportionate impact among racial and ethnic minority populations, is another example of these enduring health disparities.

The health of large numbers of people can be improved in ways that can be sustained over time by establishing policies that positively influence social and economic conditions and conditions that support changes in individual behavior. Understanding the sources and consequences of health disparities will help us better understand and internalize the importance of self-care.

Social determinants of health (SDOH) have a major impact on health, well-being, and quality of life as do physical determinants that include natural environments, such as green space (e.g., trees and grass) or weather (e.g., climate change). The Department of Health and Human Services groups the social determinants into five domains—economic stability, healthcare (access and quality), education (access and quality), environment (neighborhood and built), and community.[1]

Economic stability connects financial resources (income, cost of living, socioeconomic status) and health. With one in ten people in the United States living in poverty, access to healthy foods, healthcare, and adequate housing is denied to many.[2] Though the employed are considered to be less likely to live in poverty and may be healthier, many do not earn enough to afford what they need to be healthy. Those with disabilities, injuries, or other conditions are limited in their abilities to work.

The healthcare domain links access and quality with people's understanding of health services (primary care, health insurance coverage) and their own health literacy. Shekinah Fashaw-Walters of the University of Minnesota stated that home health agencies with high proportions of Black patients, and those located in low-income neighborhoods, are more likely to be of lower and unrated quality.[3] Care from low qualified home health agencies may result in increased adverse outcomes and is indicative of multiple levels of systemic racism.

Patricia Homan of Florida State University and Tyson Brown of Duke University concluded that reduced access to healthcare access is one of several results of Black voter suppression, along with community living and working conditions.[4]

The direct link between education and health and well-being is shown when children who struggle with math and reading tend to be less likely to graduate from high school or go to college, which means they are less likely to get jobs with sufficient pay and are more likely to have health problems like heart disease, diabetes, and depression. The stress of living in poverty can even affect brain development. Access to quality housing, transportation, healthy foods, and quality air and water also directly affect health and well-being.[5]

CHAPTER 6

Common Health Conditions in the Black Community

Much of the research on racism and health has been focused on personal racial experiences and shows that racism dysregulates the body by acting on stress pathways. The results are adverse health outcomes, daily stressors, and accelerated aging. This wear and tear, or weathering of the body, accumulates over time.

The trauma and oppression that the Black community endures has consequences for health and well-being. These consequences and their effects have also been well documented. Structural racism incorporates three levels of operating, the institutional, personal, and internalized levels.[1] Much of the research on racism and health has been focused on personal racial experiences and shows that racism dysregulates the body by acting on stress pathways. The results are adverse health outcomes, daily stressors, and accelerated aging. This wear and tear, or weathering of the body, accumulates over time.

Bringing attention to four prioritized racial inequity themes, with the first being systemic racism, then COVID-19, social determinants of health, and specific health outcomes, Mendez and colleagues specifically call out racism as a public health crisis.[2] Confronting this crisis is an important first step in dismantling systems of oppression that affect health and well-being and that contribute to health inequities.

We will take a closer look at several major health concerns in the Black community in this chapter.

Asthma

Asthma, a common chronic illness in which the lungs' bronchial tubes become swollen, constricted, or blocked, affects almost 339 million people worldwide and causes about 420,000 deaths. More than 19 million American adults, 7.7% of the United States population, have asthma. The global costs are high.[3] The condition is a common public health problem.[4]

Asthma has several causes: extrinsic (triggered by allergens), intrinsic (triggered by upper respiratory infections, air pollution, emotional stress, smoke, exercise, exposure to cold), occupational, drug-induced, or induced by exercise. The social/community, environmental, economic, educational, and healthcare domains can influence the occurrence of asthma.

According to 2017 Centers for Disease Prevention and Control numbers, Black adults have a higher prevalence of asthma than White and Hispanic adults. They also have higher death rates due to severe asthma, with three times the chances of having severe asthma. Black children are more often diagnosed with asthma than White children and they experience higher asthma-related illness, hospitalization, and death.[5]

In the general United States population, 40% of all adults have uncontrolled asthma and the disease is uncontrolled in 92% of the people that have severe asthma. While regular use of inhaled corticosteroids is safe for uncontrolled asthma and could prevent hospitalization and death associated with the disease, Blacks have the lowest adherence to using inhaled corticosteroids. The nonadherence could be partly due to misbeliefs about managing asthma and using inhaled corticosteroids as treatment, which negatively affects asthma outcomes.[6]

Breathing practices (pranayama), such as diaphragmatic breathing, have been used to treat people with asthma.[7,8] The practices can cultivate stress resilience by calming the parasympathetic nervous system, the calming part of the nervous system.[9] *Pranayama*, a Sanskrit word that means breath of life/vital energy (*prana*) and expansion/regulation (*ayama*), is one of the eight limbs of ashtanga yoga as introduced in Part 1.[10] Breathing slowly and deeply causes the airways to dilate and could possibly be helpful in its effect on asthma. This particular breathing practice is often included in pranayama and during many yoga postures (asanas) by linking breathing to movements, reducing the breathing rate.[11] Research indicates that yoga and meditation can benefit asthma due to tidal volume (the amount of air moved in and out of the lungs during each breath), breathing rate, and muscle relaxation improvements.[12]

Alzheimer's and dementia

L. L. Barnes reports that Alzheimer's disease and related dementia affects almost 6 million Americans with one in eight Americans 65 years of age and older being affected.[13] While both Alzheimer's disease and dementia affect older adults, neither is a normal part of aging. Dementia is a syndrome caused by loss in memory, thinking, behavior, and the ability to do the daily activities of living. Alzheimer's is a progressive disease that has symptoms of dementia that gradually worsen over time. As the United States population continues to age, it is estimated that more than 13 million in the United States will have Alzheimer's disease by 2050. Marginalized communities are at the highest risk and research indicates that older Black Americans are disproportionately affected. Black Americans are twice as likely to develop Alzheimer's disease and related dementias than the White population.[14]

Blacks are also more often diagnosed at later stages, resulting in an increased prevalence of chronic disease for conditions such as cardiovascular disease, stroke, and diabetes. Lifestyle choice for nutrition and exercise and social determinants of health also contribute to this inconsistent likelihood and risk among the Black community. Conditions such as diabetes and cardiovascular conditions that are significantly influenced by lifestyle are associated with higher risk for Alzheimer's disease and related dementias (AD/ADRD). According to the study by Barnes mentioned above, a number of theories indicate that racial disparities in ADRD at older ages are the result of a cumulative effect of social determinants of health disparities over a lifetime.

Even though there is a high prevalence of ADRD in the Black community, it has proven to be challenging to conduct research on the conditions that affect African Americans.[15] Some researchers put the burden on the Black community by stating that it is difficult to access racial/ethnic minorities and hard to contact people who are willing to participate in Alzheimer's disease and related dementia research. Past research incidences have led to distrust of the clinical research field. The "medical discovery" project, the US Public Health Service Syphilis Study at Tuskegee, the cloning of Henrietta Lacks' cells, radiation exposure, and experimental surgeries conducted on enslaved Black people have reinforced mistrust in research and prolonged inequitable healthcare systems.

Underrepresentation of Black people in ADRD clinical research is evident as well as in research for other conditions that include stroke and cardiovascular disease. In the case of ADRD particularly, lack of inclusion of older people in the Black community in clinical research makes it difficult to understand why the burden of this condition is so prevalent among Black Americans. A study by Shaw and colleagues indicated that successful recruitment is possible through partnership with organizations that serve the Black community. These community partners are cultural gatekeepers and help to improve recruitment and education and to reduce mistrust toward clinical research.

Spirituality is an important part of Black American culture, and research by the Alzheimer's Research and Prevention Foundation (ARPF) includes spiritual fitness as one of its four pillars for the prevention of ADRD.[16] The other three pillars are diet and supplements, stress management, and exercise. Yoga is a strategy for improving cognitive function and psychological outcomes. ARPF is conducting research to study lifestyle and Alzheimer's prevention, therapeutic benefits of yoga therapy on subjective cognitive decline, mild cognitive impairment, and Alzheimer's prevention, the merger of yoga/meditation research and technology, and spiritual fitness and Alzheimer's prevention. In one study, a daily 12-minute kirtan kriya practice over eight weeks resulted in improved cognitive functioning for both the person that had Alzheimer's disease as well as the caregiver.[17] Kirtan (praise, sing) kriya (act, action) is a meditation practice that includes repeating a phrase (mantra) that symbolizes birth, life, death, and rebirth.

Obesity and overweight

Factors such as race, location, gender, and education affect patterns of obesity, a public health concern and a growing source of morbidity and mortality in the United States, especially among the non-Hispanic Black population. Among non-Hispanic Black women, higher income does not protect against obesity, unlike other demographic groups. The frequency of obesity also impacts the incidences of stroke and cardiovascular disease. Adiposity data on Black women result from measurable and difficult to measure social determinants that affect health disparities. Behavioral weight loss intervention research shows that Black women lose less weight and that they have body positivity at higher weight levels. While this is healthy psychologically, it can decrease motivation for losing weight.[18] There can be a disconnect between a positive body image and poor health outcomes.[19]

Obesity and sedentary lifestyles can also affect the management of asthma and are associated with more increased occurrences of asthma and a decreased quality of life.[20] There is also a medication burden associated with treating asthma. Lifestyle interventions can be adjunct treatments. Individuals with asthma are less likely to exercise than those that do not have asthma, resulting in more severe cases.

Whether or not the terms overweight and obese are derogatory terms is still debatable. Rather than assigning obesity to who a person is, obesity is a condition like a person having heart or respiratory conditions, among other conditions. The causes of obesity are modifiable (physical activity, healthy diet) and non-modifiable (genetics, metabolism, developmental conditions). The social determinants of health (SDOH) also influence making healthy decisions. Because SDOHs and psychosocial factors influence approximately 80% of poor health outcomes, medical care cannot singularly change the health outcome. Underlying issues that lead to overweight and obesity can also be addressed through prevention and treatment.[21]

In Prince George's County in southern Maryland, Black women are significantly impacted by obesity. A study by Jovonni Spinner shows obesity leads to poor physical and mental health and decreased social well-being, and financially strains the healthcare system. Prince George's County is an educated, middle to high income area where Black women have difficulty managing their weight.[22] According to Spinner, a researcher at Morgan State University in Baltimore, Maryland, social and cultural factors and social networks impact the weight of these Black women. These social and cultural factors include income, family network, peer network, and living in the county.[23]

Prince George's County, outside of Washington, DC, is an affluent suburb where 60% of the residents are Black. Half of these Black residents are women with a median age of 38. Over 46% of these women earn more than $75,000 a year (higher than the 2018 national average), 68% own their homes, 39% have college degrees, and 28% attended some college or trade school. Despite this affluence Black women have higher rates of overweight and obesity than their White counterparts. This data aligns with state and national trends. These higher rates of overweight and obesity, observed across income and education levels, may suggest that other determinants of health impact weight status among Black women. More research is needed to explore the health behaviors of middle to high income Black women and how social and cultural factors impact overweight and obesity.[24]

This study was a snapshot of a small group of 15 Black women that represented their unique perspectives, some part of the same social network.[25] Participants in the Spinner study stated that Black culture is more accepting of larger and curvy body types, reinforcing a positive body image and supporting less focus on achieving an ideal body mass index (BMI), a measure of a person's weight in relation to height. (To determine BMI, multiply weight in pounds and divide that by the square of height in inches.[26] A BMI greater than 25 is considered overweight, and obese is a BMI greater than 30.)

The National Institute of Health (NIH) now uses BMI to define underweight, normal weight, overweight, and obese rather than height and weight charts, as does the World Health Organization.[27] The BMI classifications are also used to determine risks for chronic diseases like hypertension, diabetes, depression, and cancer. Waist-to-hip ratio, percentage of body or visceral fat, and waist circumference are additional methods that can be used to determine obesity. Though considerable importance is put on using BMI rather than height and weight tables, the BMI measurement has limitations, particularly for evaluating people who could have excess body fat (adiposity) and for understanding the diversity of obesity. BMI does not indicate how fat is distributed, which could be a marker for greater cardiometabolic disease and cancer risks. A better choice could be to measure the accumulation of visceral fat in the abdominal area and waist circumference, and the use of imaging techniques. Waist circumference is a better marker of obesity-related health risk.[28]

Uncontrolled obesity and overweight can lead to chronic health conditions that include cardiovascular disease, metabolic disease, and mental health concerns that affect quality of life and financially strain the healthcare system. People that live with obesity and overweight can also face stigma, discrimination, and in some cases social isolation.

Cultural and social factors associated with food, stress, and religion come into play when making weight-based decisions. Social cognitive theory explains that, with regards to our health, our decision-making ability is influenced by individual experiences, the external environment, and the actions of others. Positive changes in health behavior then require social support, building self-efficacy, and observational learning.[29]

Culture can also influence personal views of health and wellness. Tradition and history result in varying approaches toward eating and physical activity habits. In Black culture there is a spirit of collectivism and family and friends play a central role. Historically, generational oppression led to disenfranchisement and economic and health disparities.[30]

While income and the high cost of being healthy were noted as general issues, these more affluent women could buy what they needed to be healthy, such as exercise equipment, high-end groceries, gym memberships, and personal trainers; some participants stated that if they were not financially stable, they would not be able to shop at high-end grocers, buy juicers and blenders, and buy exercise equipment.

The women in the Spinner study were concerned about how Black women can be negatively portrayed in the media. Most of the women in the study wanted to change generational habits and become healthier for themselves and to set positive examples for their children. Programs that mainly focus on diets and physical modifications do not sufficiently address how decisions are made.[31] Creating self-care practices that also incorporate ethical yoga philosophy can prove to be a pathway for resisting societal pressure to look or act a certain way as Black women and men. Obesity is also a factor in many diseases that include diabetes mellitus, hypertension, stroke, cardiovascular disease,[32] and asthma.[33]

A growing body of research shows that the risk of obesity and metabolic syndrome is decreased with physical activity. The popularity of yoga as a form of physical activity is growing, but other yoga practices that include relaxation, breathing exercises, and meditation are also beneficial. The yoga postures (asanas) provide physical activity and stress reduction.[34] They also calm the nervous system. Other limbs of yoga such as restraints (yama), observances (niyama), withdrawal of the senses (focused awareness), and concentration (dharana) can also be helpful. The effects of yoga on obesity, overweight, and metabolic syndrome are connected to behavior change, immune status, and nervous system regulation.

Yoga can potentially reduce negative body image and promote positive body image. According to research by Webb and colleagues, body positivity involves positively connecting with the body, appreciating body functions, self-care, expressing the body's desires, and seeing the body as subjective and based on personal feelings rather than those of others.[35] Positive body image involves satisfaction with body appearance and function, body experiences, and coping with challenges related to having a healthy body image. Yoga practitioners tend to focus on how the body feels internally more than how it looks externally.

Cardiovascular disease

Cardiovascular disease (CVD) affects many Americans 60 years of age and older. The American Heart Association identifies indicators of biological and behavioral domains to describe ideal cardiovascular health. The biological indicators are blood pressure, glucose, cholesterol, and body mass index (BMI). The behavioral indicators are diet, physical activity, and smoking. Research shows that maintaining cardiovascular health is fundamental to healthy aging, lower mortality associated with cardiovascular disease, reduced physical disability, and less cognitive decline as we age.[36]

Epidemiological studies show that Black adults score lower than White adults on all components of cardiovascular health except for lipid profiles, blood tests for fatty acids like cholesterol and triglycerides. (Epidemiology is the study and analysis of disease within a population and the cornerstone of public health.)[37] As cardiovascular health improves, there is a decrease in age-related disease and death later in life. The disparities in cardiovascular health can be seen at the intersection of marginalization with Black adults tending to have lower cardiovascular health. Black women score the lowest in cardiovascular health followed by Black men, White men, and White women, respectively.[38]

These racial disparities may begin early in life because the gap is also evident among children. There is a possible inference that early life adversity (ELA), discrimination, and socioeconomic status (SES) are likely reasons. While there has been little investigation into a correlation between life factors and cardiovascular health, race and gender disparities in cardiovascular disease have been well documented.[39]

Studies based on the National Health and Nutrition Examination Survey and the Coronary Artery Risk Development in Young Adults study indicate that among White women and men, White women have better cardiovascular health, and Black women and men have similar cardiovascular health. The higher cardiovascular health of White women is attributed to the protective effects of endogenous estrogens, especially before menopause. That is not the case for Black adults. Why? One hypothesis is that multi-level social categorization, along with race/ethnicity, gender, and age, forms a system of oppression for the marginalized and that could be associated with adverse health outcomes. Black women are at the bottom of racial and gender social hierarchies, they are impacted by more obstacles to ideal cardiovascular health, and there is a greater chance that they have fewer resources to respond to more of life's adversities and social and material difficulties. While Black men are considered to have a subordinate racial hierarchy, they are privileged in the gender hierarchy.

Cardiovascular health may be impacted by early life stress or traumatic experiences due to altered physiological structure and function. This, in turn, can negatively impact development cognitively and socially and increase the chance of embracing unhealthy behaviors and lifestyles. These early life experiences, such as maltreatment, may lead to lower education levels in young adulthood and lower economic attainment in midlife, and involve more discrimination, which is associated with elevated allostatic load.[40]

According to Khalsa and colleagues psychosocial stress and adverse emotional states are risk factors for hypertension, stroke, other cardiovascular conditions, and cardiovascular mortality.[41] Evidence shows that yoga can reduce stress and support improvements in cardiovascular response and recovery by balancing the autonomic nervous system and decreasing allostatic load, the cumulative effect of chronic stress and life events on the human body.[42] When the challenges of life exceed a person's ability to manage those life events the result is allostatic load.

Diabetes mellitus

Diabetes mellitus, the seventh leading cause of death in the United States, substantially contributes to damaging physical health. It affects the nation's economic health also. Among all chronic diseases, diabetes is ranked the highest in healthcare costs and public spending. It is a premorbid condition[43] and a global health problem that is prevalent among Blacks, though questions still remain about the genetic risks associated with the condition.[44]

Due to racial and socioeconomic disparities, the human and economic costs associated with diabetes are borne by the burden of increased disease in underserved communities.[45] Diabetes mellitus is associated with lower socioeconomic status that includes education, income, and occupation.[46]

Within the concept of physical health, for some adults diagnosed with diabetes who received care in community health centers, housing instability could be as high as 30%. And housing instability was associated with more trips to emergency departments and hospitalizations. For those that lived in walkable neighborhoods and with greater access to green spaces there were fewer incidences of diabetes and better overall health.[47]

Even though there have been improvements in the treatment of diabetes mellitus, racial disparities still affect diabetes outcomes.[48] During the period 1999 to 2018 Black adults diagnosed with diabetes mellitus were less likely to reach clinical and quality targets than White adults. Black adults were also 1.5 to 2.5 times more likely to suffer with the complications of diabetes mellitus like diabetic retinopathy, lower limb amputation, major cardiovascular disease, stroke, and end stage renal disease than White adults. Additionally they are three times more likely to be hospitalized for uncontrolled diabetes and short-term complications.[49]

A 2003 report by the Institute of Medicine, entitled *Unequal Treatment*, reported that healthcare, as one of the social determinants of health, contributes to lower socioeconomic status of racial/ethnic groups. These inequities are perpetuated by implicit racial bias that influences attitudes, communication, and clinical decision making.[50] Diabetes is disproportionally prevalent in Indigenous peoples of America (15.9%), Black (13.2%), Hispanic (12.8%), and Asian Americans (9%). The condition affects 7.6% of White Americans. Approximately 90% of all diabetes cases are classified as type 2 diabetes. This type of diabetes is distinguished by hyperglycemia due to pancreatic beta cell dysfunction with a decrease in insulin secretion and insulin resistance.[51]

Type 2 diabetes susceptibility is due to age, obesity, family history, and ethnicity. The condition can also include kidney disease. Mechanisms of yoga can decrease the negative impact of stress and neuroendocrine status, and inflammatory responses.[52] They can also change the nervous system response from sympathetic to parasympathetic, feasibly through vagus nerve (10th cranial nerve) stimulation.

Hypertension

Hypertension, the silent killer, is prevalent in the Black population. Hypertension is called a silent killer because people that have high blood pressure may not be aware that they have the condition until their blood vessels and major organs are damaged. The only way to know if blood pressure is elevated is to measure it. But individuals that have hypertension are often told that hypertension is affected by behaviors that they can self-manage.[53]

The reason there is a prevalence in Blacks is often attributed to their environment, psychosocial stressors, socioeconomic conditions, and behavior. Substantial obstacles to controlling blood pressure are physical activity recommendations, diet, and adhering to prescribed medications. Nonadherence to these controllable obstacles occurs in everyday life. Strategies to include more physical activity, self-care activities, and physical and social environments to practice the strategies happen at the individual level.[54]

Hypertension develops earlier in the lives of Blacks. It is often accompanied by higher cardiovascular disease risk when compared to other racial or ethnic groups. There is also a higher prevalence in Blacks of higher death rates associated with the condition. When comparing gender, Black women are found to have the higher rates of physical inactivity, overweight/obesity, and stroke and heart failure prevalence. This indicates that Black women have an even greater need to modify lifestyle in order to maintain blood pressure control.[55] Black women have the highest prevalence for hypertension in the world. The prevention and management effort to control high blood pressure appears to be ineffective. Educating Black women and calling out the importance of a commitment to self-care is critical.[56]

There is a standardized evidence-based intervention for managing chronic disease called the Chronic Disease Self-Management Program. When used, the program is said to help improve and sustain health outcomes. The program accomplishes this by helping patients adhere to medication, improve health literacy, improving communication between the patient and the provider, decreasing emergency room visits, and reducing hospitalizations: in other words, helping patients to actively participate in their care. They learn, practice, and implement self-care within a supportive environment and receive feedback on how they are progressing.[57]

Several practices of yoga, lifestyle and culture, diet, and movement/

physical exercise have been proven to improve blood pressure.[58] These practices contribute to lowering blood pressure via the mechanisms of cognitive top-down regulation and physical body related bottom-up regulation.

Mental health

In 2021 the American Psychological Association (APA) issued a statement about its historical involvement in racial discrimination and stated that it is now committed to health equity and ending systemic racism against people of color in America.[59] Racial discrimination is one of the ways that racism affects health.[60] Marginalized individuals are more vulnerable to mental illness due to higher rates of poverty and other socioeconomic factors and are therefore less likely to seek treatment from primary care providers[61] or to take advantage of prescription drugs for mental illness.[62]

The APA defines mental health as "a state of mind characterized by emotional well-being, good behavioral adjustment, relative freedom from anxiety and disabling symptoms, and a capacity to establish constructive relationships and cope with the ordinary demands and stresses of life."[63] Chronic stressors can affect physical and mental health. The stress associated with navigating a life of poverty can even impact cognitive ability, performing tasks, and mistrust when dealing with healthcare providers, resulting in limited health outcomes.[64]

Repeated exposure to stressors such as racism during a life span increases the allostatic load and compromises health. Allostatic load measures physiological dysregulation caused by chronic stress on the body.[65] Primary allostasis moderators are the hormones cortisol, adrenaline, and interleukins and, over time, sustained overload of these hormones can compromise health.[66]

A Surgeon General report indicates that cultural and racial disparities in mental healthcare have not improved.[67] Whites are twice as likely as Blacks to seek mental healthcare. When Black people are diagnosed with a mental health disorder, they are reluctant to obtain treatment, continuing the mental healthcare disparities.[68]

Black people are less likely to receive mental health services and less likely to access these services in general healthcare or inpatient settings. In the United States, integrating behavioral health in primary care is considered essential and across races, there was greater improvement in mental health when it was given by primary care providers. Black people mostly received mental health treatment from mental health professionals. They also experienced poorer outcomes. Added to the dilemma, Blacks are less likely to have a primary doctor. A study by Henry and colleagues found that Black people were more likely to receive treatment from mental health providers with varying outcomes.[69] Those that sought care from mental health providers experienced less improvement than those receiving care from primary care providers. One reason for this may be that those who see mental health providers begin treatment with a worse mental health status.

In other words, those that receive treatment from primary care providers have the highest improvement as compared to those that receive care from mental health providers.[70] In a primary care setting patients have milder forms of distress and have greater improvement in mental component scores. The three mental health components are cognitive health, emotional health, and behavioral health. Those who see mental health providers may have more severe and persistent mental illness and experience lower changes in mental component scores.

Poor health literacy is one of the barriers to receiving mental health treatment. Other barriers are geographic and financial, as well as attitudes toward mental health treatment.[71] Treatment efficacy can be impacted by a willingness to seek help, talk to professionals, and believe that treatment helps.

Of the three leading reasons for disability, mental illness such as depression and substance abuse cost more than $180 billion for treatment and support. The direct cost of lost productivity, quality of life, housing unpredictability, and the need for social support services cannot be measured, but it is expected to increase.[72]

Scientific research indicates that mental health is declining for minority youth. While suicide is the eighth leading cause of death for individuals aged 10 to 34, it is the second leading cause of death overall. While Indigenous peoples of America have the highest rate of suicide, it is the third leading cause of death for Black Americans between the ages of 15 and 24.[73]

The meditation component of yoga and other yogic practices can help deep relaxation, positive changes in attitude, improved self-regulation, stabilizing emotions, and improved stress resilience.[74] Yoga practices can also improve neuropsychological risk profiles along with cognition, relaxation, and improved positive outlook.

Pain

The consequences of pain impact health and the quality of life. Relative to Whites, Black Americans are undertreated for pain. In some cases, this treatment can be attributed to inaccurate beliefs about biological differences (such as Blacks having thicker skin or blood that coagulates quicker), contributing to racial disparities and underprescription of medications for Black patients. Racial and ethnic minority populations receive treatment for pain less frequently when compared to Whites despite the rapid growth of attention to the pain field in the past 20 years. Could this be due to not having healthcare access, or that Black patients' pain is not recognized, therefore not treated? In a study by Hoffman and colleagues physicians underestimated the pain that Black patients experience.[75]

Highlighting the growing awareness of disparities in pain treatment, the Joint Commission on Accreditation of Hospitals and Health Care Organizations (JACHO) identified pain relief as a measure of quality pain care and that people have a right to adequate pain care.[76] The National Institutes of Health (NIH) defines health disparities as "differences in the incidence, prevalence, mortality, and burden of disease and other adverse health conditions existing among specific population groups in the United States."[77] Disparities in providing pain care to African Americans occur in the following areas:

1. How pain is perceived.

2. Communicating the presence of pain to healthcare providers.

3. Healthcare provider assessment of pain intensity.

4. Administration of pain relievers by emergency healthcare providers.[78]

Differences in pain treatment is a priority for cancer pain research. In a study that looked at centers that cared for predominantly racial and ethnic minority patients, patients were undertreated and undermedicated.[79]

Chronic pain, a global health problem, affects millions of people.[80] Individuals that experience chronic pain as part of their daily lives look for ways to cope with it. The connection between pain, emotion, and cognition makes mind–body therapies such as yoga and meditation effective and the practices can potentially help practitioners develop strategies for dealing with pain and in some cases help alleviate pain.

As a chronic condition, pain is complex and experienced differently by each person. Mind–body therapies like meditation and yoga may help by regulating cognitive and emotional responses. Negative memories and emotions can cause an increase in pain and a positive response could decrease it.

COVID-19

As of June 2020, coronavirus disease 2019 (COVID-19) had affected over 8 million people and had killed more than 450,000 people from 200 countries. At one time there was a "we are all in this together" sentiment that did not translate to ethnic impartiality. There were overwhelming racial disparities in the United States. COVID-19 disproportionately infected and killed non-Whites.[81]

The Centers for Disease Control and Prevention (CDC) determined that while Blacks were only 13% of the United States population, they comprised a third of hospitalizations across 14 states that were analyzed. Blacks were 18% of the population of those areas. According to a Washington Post report the infection rates of predominantly Black counties were three times higher than those of counties that were predominantly White. Seventy percent of the COVID-19 deaths in Louisiana were Black. That is twice the 32% Black population in the state. In New York state (excluding New York City) 17% of the COVID-19 deaths were Black, though Blacks were only 9% of the population.[82]

Inadequate access to medical care and food, crowded living conditions, and reliance on public transportation have been linked to health disparities for decades. There are also disproportionately high incidences of health conditions such as diabetes mellitus, hypertension, obesity, asthma, and cardiovascular disease in these same populations.[83] Additionally, constant low-level inflammation is characteristic of chronic disease.[84] These all merge to present the complex influences of comorbid risk.[85]

The CDC identified these health conditions, along with chronic lung disease, chronic kidney disease and dialysis, immunocompromising conditions, morbid obesity (40 or greater BMI), smoking, and being at least 65 years old, as predisposing these individuals to severe COVID-19. A significant number of the individuals hospitalized for COVID-19 had one or more of these conditions.[86]

The pandemic put a spotlight on the deeply-rooted healthcare inequities. There was evidence in the first month of the COVID outbreak that there were going to be higher rates of hospitalization and mortality for Black patients as compared to White patients. The rate was 1.6 times higher for Black residents and 1.4 times higher for Hispanic residents in New York City.[87]

Interestingly, there were no differences for those younger than 19 years of age. The increase in disparities as people age could indicate that over time the compounding effect of social determinants leads to decreases in health and increased susceptibility to unfavorable COVID-19 related outcomes.[88]

A commitment to resolve structural racism and a vision of improved health equity are imperatives. The pandemic made what is already apparent clearer. Health disparities will not improve without a better understanding of the racial disparities associated with COVID-19 nor will this community be better positioned for future medical crises. There are multiple reasons for the health risks in Black communities in the United States. Research in England also tells that there is more to the story of comorbidity and the social determinant of health relationship to disease risk and mortality in vulnerable populations.[89]

Black women

Throughout the study of health disparities in the Black community, the dilemma of Black women being at the bottom of the scale continually emerges, though there have been improvements in health in the last 50 years. Despite this progress, Black women continue to have shorter life expectancies compared to other women, have higher rates of maternal mortality, and disproportionately suffer with chronic conditions like cardiovascular disease and obesity. The health outcomes are experienced within the context of their social conditions, and the burden of the chronic conditions are a reflection of structural inequities that are experienced throughout the course of these women's lives. This is not a singular incident.[90]

The health of Black women is grounded in slavery. White slave holders considered enslaved Black women to be property to be used for economic gain. Their bodies were abused and they were forced to reproduce without regard for their self-agency and health. When the gynecology specialty was created in the 1850s Black women were the targets of immoral experimentation that still continues in the 21st century. "Black women are at the center of a public health emergency."[91]

Black women comprise a diverse ethnic group from different cultures. They are about 7% of the United States population and 13.6% of all women in the United States. Even though they are generally younger at 36 years old than the 40 years of United States women overall, they have a higher occurrence of health conditions (heart disease, stroke, cancer, diabetes, obesity, stress, and maternal morbidities). The life expectancy at birth is three years less than for White females and the mortality rate is higher for Black infants, particularly infants born to Black female teens.

As Black women age, health disparities increase as socioeconomic disadvantages and racist experiences increase.[92] The telomeres of Black women of 49–55 years indicate that Black women are biologically 7.5 years older than White women. (Telomeres are DNA structures at the ends of chromosomes; they are markers for aging.)

Black women are incredibly resilient and must aggressively advocate for themselves in order to receive quality healthcare and not merely survive the legacy and theory that poor health outcomes are a measure of the health of Black women.[93] Gail Parker, PhD, explains that the "Sojourner Syndrome," a gender specific strategy to weather any storm, to be strong at all times, suppress physical and emotional pain, and succeed at all costs, is a coping strategy used by Black women.[94] This coping strategy for resisting adversity and oppression exacts a toll on health that can be influenced by practicing ease through restorative yoga practices.

Conclusion

Health inequities confronting Black Americans complicate the presence of multiple pre-existing health conditions and perpetuate the disproportionate number of deaths caused by COVID-19.[95] More than 180,000 COVID-related deaths occurred in the United States. While all racial/ethnic groups were affected, most were Black Americans. The social determinants of health (socioeconomic, environmental, education, and healthcare) and chronic stress combined can change the body's biological makeup and increase risks for chronic disease. Chronic psychological stress caused by an increase in cortisol is associated with chronic inflammatory disease. Other pre-existing conditions not related to stress are also mechanisms for inflammatory diseases. The intersection between environment (SDOH and stress), comorbidity, and genes points us to a space that is a hot bed for poor outcomes such as disproportionate COVID-19 deaths in the Black community.

Health risk in the Black community is influenced by multiple factors. Research in England indicates that pre-existing disease and the social determinants of health may not account for all health risks in underserved populations.[96] Add biopsychosocial factors and persistent low-level inflammation could be a leading factor for most chronic health outcomes. Psychological stress is also identified as a risk factor for cardiovascular conditions and other conditions that impact Black communities.

Racism affects all of us, whether we are aware of it or not. It affects our ability to know, relate to, and value one another. Systemically, it is one of the biggest obstacles to solving the challenges we face in our communities.[97]

Fanny Brewster, PhD, recalls in *Archetypal Grief: Slavery's Legacy of Intergenerational Child Loss* that philosophically there is a belief among African people "that there is no separation of mind and body. The body remembers long after the mind has forgotten what it has seen or heard." [98] The body tells a story. This position has become more evident recently as we see the development of somatic psychology as an area of professional practice for psychologists.[99]

"We know grief and suffering because it is a defining aspect of being human... If grief is possible, so is resiliency."[100] Black people are intergenerationally still living the suffering of slavery and cultural trauma. Healing from race-based trauma is a path of restoring wholeness. Brewster states that revisiting the African Holocaust as many times as we can tolerate is called for to view and revise how the Black community changes perspectives for peaceful relationships with each other. We can also change our relationships with ourselves. "Who-we-have-been need not be the future-selves-we-are-becoming."[101] Yoga provides an opportunity to move toward personal healing.

Three components of ashtanga yoga involve controlling breath (pranayama), physical activity (postures/asana), and relaxation (meditation/savasana). By focusing on controlling the breath, moving through and holding postures, and meditation, yoga can increase a practitioner's attention to bodily sensation and to being present to the moment, which can contribute to a presence in our activities. Yoga interventions and mindfulness may be helpful with diabetes mellitus,[102] obesity,[103] cardiovascular disease, mental health,[104] pain,[105] and COVID-19.[106,107]

Yoga researchers are increasingly more interested in exploring how the mechanisms of yoga correlate with its psychophysiological effects. According to Raveendran and colleagues this work requires a close look at the function of yoga to understand how yoga can be an intravention and way to explore within, in addition to being an intervention.[108] Gail Parker points out in *Restorative Yoga for Ethnic and Race-Based Stress and Trauma* that, while yoga and meditation can reduce stress and anxiety, people who need the practices often cannot experience the benefits of yoga and meditation: without "the necessary tools to address emotional discomfort in a constructive, non-defensive, non-confrontational, non-avoidant way, opportunities for deeper understanding and connection are missed. Yoga offers us a starting point."[109]

PART III

DEMYSTIFYING YOGA IN THE BLACK COMMUNITY

This section discusses the cultural and religious taboos of practicing yoga in the Black community. A comparative alignment of yoga philosophy and principles and Black American cultural and religious practices explores the tangible aspects of these healing modalities to support the health and well-being of the Black community.

CHAPTER 7

Do Black Folk Practice Yoga?

Yoga is a universal manner of personal inquiry that explores our collective question "What does it mean to be human?"

According to the Centers for Disease Control and Prevention's National Center for Health Statistics' 2017 Health Survey on the Use of CAM Among Racial Groups in the United States, 9.3% of Blacks surveyed practice yoga, an increase from 2.5% of those surveyed 15 years earlier in 2002.[1] Of those, 13.5% also practice meditation. Although more Black folks are practicing yoga today, the majority of African Americans do not. Why?

In our experience of offering a practice of yoga in the Black community, participants often declined stating because they are Christian (or "because of my religion") they cannot practice yoga. Exploring the tenets of Christianity as adapted by African Americans, deviation from the faith may occur if one "worships" other than the Holy Trinity—Father (God), the son (Jesus Christ), and the Holy Ghost. Both the Old and New Testaments of the Holy Bible include multiple warnings within their books and verses about worshiping idols, especially those created by man's own hands. Interpretations of both Old and New Testaments declare the presence of one God, and the New Testament's interpretation is that there is solely one way to get to know God and higher consciousness and that is through the teaching of Jesus Christ.

Understanding these foundational tenets of the Christian faith, it stands to reason that a practice associated with multiple deities and other uncommon rituals would be off-putting. But this is due to a misunderstanding of yoga—a misunderstanding that "yoga" is associated *as* either Hindu and/or Buddhist religions that do reverence idols and deities within their traditions. Common definitions published in US English language dictionaries perpetuate this misunderstanding by defining yoga as "a Hindu discipline aimed at training the consciousness for a state of perfect spiritual insight and tranquility."[2] Although both these religious faiths as well as others such as Jainism, Sikhism, and Sufism employ yoga philosophy and practices and thus their mystical cosmologies are often linked with yoga, these religions are not "yoga."

Yoga is a universal manner of personal inquiry that explores our collective question "What does it mean to be human?" Like the Christian teachings of Jesus Christ that establishes a spiritual path toward understanding one's eternal soul, Jesus' invitation to this path is to "Take my yoke upon you, and learn of me, for I am gentle and lowly in heart, and ye shall find rest unto your souls" (Matthew 11:29).[3] Yoga too is a practice of "yoking" or joining onto a journey of self-inquiry that through a disciplined system will elevate one's consciousness and alleviate the sufferings of the heart, mind, and soul.

Although the origin of yoga predates its familiar 6000-year history, evidence of humans' interest in cultivating their understanding of the universe and consciousness is found in centuries-earlier hieroglyphic drawings and in ancient written texts worldwide. The ethical principles and way of life of yoga are the basis for spirituality in Indian society and greatly influence the South Asian geographic area and populations. Here yoga "refers to that enormous body of spiritual values, attitudes, precepts, and techniques that have been developed in India over at least five millennia and that may be regarded as the very foundation of the ancient Indian civilization."[4]

These yogic ethical principles gleaned in various religious texts such as the Vedas and Upanishads evolved into formal religious practices such as Hinduism, Buddhism, and Jainism. As highlighted in Part I and will be discussed in Part IV, Patanjali codified a systematic approach to seeking knowledge in the Yoga Sutras.[5] Patanjali's yogic system, ashtanga yoga, weaves a sequential formula for obtaining enlightenment. The practices of the eight limbs of yoga (ashtanga) as classified in Patanjali's Yoga Sutras leads the practitioner yogi to live life through righteous action: kriya yoga.

The value and importance of the religious life in the Black community cannot be overestimated. According to the U.S. Religious Landscape Survey, conducted in 2014 by the Pew Research Center's Forum on

Religion & Public Life, 79% of Black Americans consider themselves Christian, with 83% expressing absolute certainty in the belief in God.[6] Fifty-three percent of Black Christians follow historically Black Protestant affiliations. Three percent of Black Americans surveyed embrace non-Christian faiths, 1% consider themselves either Buddhist, Hindu, or Jewish, and 2% consider themselves Muslim. Eighteen percent of Black Americans surveyed declare no affiliation with a religious faith.

The Christian church in particular "has served as a major institutional foundation of African American spiritual and community life."[7] During enslavement, the church—as a body—provided the sole source for Blacks to congregate as one community and fellowship together. In many instances the church was the first school of education for Blacks, who learned to read and write through the use of the Holy Bible. Enslaved African acculturation as "African Americans" was solidified through religious life that evolved into the various Black Protestant denominations (e.g., Black Baptist, African Methodist Episcopal, Holiness/Pentecostal) that continue to flourish today.

Religious practice in the Black community is vast and celebrated in a variety of interpretations. In Chapter 2 we reference the impact on enslaved African spiritual customs with the forced conversion to Christian doctrine. "Christianity was largely viewed [by Whites] as an instrument of social control, to produce 'obedient and docile' slaves."[8] However, the importance of maintaining one's indigenous faith led to the appropriation of European American-styled Christianity into African American religious values and culture. For example, it is estimated that "15–30% of Africans imported as slaves were Muslim."[9] In an autobiography of an enslaved Black Muslim in the United States written in 1851, we have the example of Christian acculturation in the life of Omar ibn Said, an educated man from Futa Toro (now known as Senegal) who was captured during tribal wars and sold into slavery.[10] Although Omar ibn Said converted to Christianity after being captured, he maintained various aspects of his Muslim faith. His autobiography *Oh ye Americans* includes passages that are transliterations of prayers and *iyats* (verses) of the Holy Qur'an, the religious scripture of the Muslim world. Omar ibn Said's autobiography includes the story of his captivity and, through sharing passages from the Holy Qur'an, he urges Americans to live and practice the faith (Christianity) that they profess and preach.

I reside in this country by reason of great necessity. Wicked men took me by violence and sold me to the Christians. We sailed a month and a half on the great sea to the place called Charleston in the Christian land. I fell into the hands of a small, weak and wicked man, who feared not God at all, nor did he read (the gospel) at all nor pray. I was afraid to remain with this a man so depraved and who committed so many crimes and I ran away. After a month our Lord God brought me forward to the hand of a good man, who fears God, and loves to do good... O ye Americans, ye people of North Carolina, have you, have you, have you, have you among you a family like this family, having so much love to God as they?[11]

Many enslaved Africans descended from indigenous matriarchal cultures and societies that influenced the role of African women in leading the newfound Christian religious life in the American diaspora. Throughout the history of matriarchal societies worldwide, a common thread of principles fortified their cultural foundation, gender equity, consensus building, and respect for all life. "Demonstratively, matriarchal societies are true societies of peace," writes anthropologist Heide Goettner-Abendroth. "They are non-violent, and their relationships lack the interpersonal, social, and economic barbarism so prevalent in patriarchal societies, especially in western civilizations."[12]

In African matriarchies, such as the Asante and Akan of West Africa, women were and are revered as the primary lineage holders of the culture—women being the natural bearers of life and thus the maintainers of future generations. Women serve as leaders of the community, give voice to all major tribal decisions, economic, social, political, and spiritual, equally with the male leadership to "generate balance in accordance with traditional conception and belief."[13] African matriarchies, much like other matriarchal societies worldwide, maintained their cohesiveness as a closed society to ward off the influence and dominance of patriarchies striving to usurp their rich culture of peace. Much of the history and traditions within matriarchies are exclusively handed down through oral tradition as a means of preserving their principles and practices.[14]

Notwithstanding, enslaved African women within the newly forming Black Christian church assumed similar leadership roles that would assure the health and well-being of the African American communities within the American enslaved culture, for instance, a non-denominational Christian "secret" society of Black women founded by enslaved Africans Annetta M. Lane and Harriet R. Taylor in 1867. As the oldest Black women's organization in the United States, the United Order of

Tents was initially organized to support Black women escape from slavery in collaboration with the Underground Railroad of enslaved Blacks seeking freedom.[15]

As an enslaved woman living in the southern state of Virginia, Annetta Lane served as a nurse for enslaved Africans as well as White slave holders and that afforded her access to both worlds and also the ability to support Black women seeking to migrate to free American states. Upon obtaining her freedom, Lane, along with her co-founder Harriet Taylor, strengthened the foundation of her work as a secret order within Black Christian church communities, organizing women to pool their creative abilities and financial resources to support their community with financial investment, housing, and healthcare, three major aspects of quality of life that the Black community was denied equal access to. The United Order of Tents provided a "tent of salvation"[16] to "most importantly, serve as affirmation of Black personhood, dignity, and independence at a time when the wider world insisted on Black inferiority."[17] Standing true to the tradition of the African matriarchal values of maintaining cohesion of the community and securing sacred knowledge by oral tradition, the United Order of Tents' secrecy assured that their work to build a free African American society would not be destroyed by the dominant culture of white supremacy.

The United Order of Tents' mission and vision states:

> We believe that it is our duty as Christians and citizens of the United States of America to do all within our power to assist in attending to the sick, to raise in the heart a fountain of purity and love such as will be a joy to the living and a source of consolation to the bereaved. We believe it is our duty to encourage the youth in seeking their highest potential, to care for the aged, respectfully bury the dead, promote sisterhood and love among ourselves and our posterity, invoking the favor and guidance of Almighty God.[18]

For over 100 years, the United Order of Tents was successfully self-sufficient in supporting the communities their membership lived and worked in. "Even today in the 21st century, the Tents operate in secret."[19] However, its membership is comprised of Black women from all social classes and "does not exclude any woman based on [her] situation in life...wealth, or...lack of wealth, prestige, or denomination."[20]

The essence of the United Order of Tents' commitment to the Black community is grounded comparatively with the ashtanga yogic limbs, yama and niyama, as evidenced by their dedication to a respect for life (*ahimsa*), insistence on upholding the dignity of all members of the Black community (*aparigraha*), and steadfast commitment to seeking the pleasure of the God they serve (*ishvara pranidhana*).

Further acculturation of Christianity within the African American religious context continued into the 20th century. During the Black civil rights movement that culminated in the 1960s, Black theologian James H. Cone focused his religious study of Christianity on a fundamental Black American principle—liberation. Cone's work was influenced by two primary spiritual political leaders of his time, Martin Luther King, Jr., a practicing Christian, and Malcolm X, a practicing Muslim. A practicing Christian, Cone identified with Martin Luther King, Jr.'s moral compass and belief in Jesus Christ. He also identified with Malcolm X's stratagem that Blacks needed to be free from the oppression of systemic racism. Through this lens and like a resurrection of enslaved Africans' adaptation of their historical conversion to Christianity, Cone believed and taught that "Christianity is essentially a religion of liberation."[21] He explored the historical records of oppressed people that are identified in Biblical text and related such histories to the oppression that African Americans are experiencing in the Western hemisphere. Cone's Black liberation theology treatise is that God is always working on the side of the oppressed and is always seeking their liberation from their oppressors.

"Black theology is a theology of liberation because it is a theology which arises from an identification with the oppressed Black of America," Cone writes in *A Black Theology of Liberation*. "[Black theology is] seeking to interpret the gospel of Jesus in the light of the Black condition. It believes that the liberation of the Black community is God's liberation."[22]

Cone also challenged the concept of God as a Caucasian figurehead since he believed that God is the God of the oppressed and Blacks in America are the oppressed people. "It is the black theology emphasis on the blackness of God that distinguishes it sharply from contemporary white views of God," writes Cone. "White religionists are not capable of perceiving the blackness of God, because their satanic whiteness is a denial of the very essence of divinity. This is why whites are finding and will continue to find the black experience a disturbing reality."[23]

A unique blend of African American cultural and spiritual practices and principles gave rise to the work of Maulana Karenga. Karenga is an ethical philosopher, teacher, and scholar of ancient Egyptian ethics, and the theory and practice of African American nationalism.[24] A prolific writer, lecturer, and activist, Karenga founded the non-profit organization, US, that is dedicated to making humanity "self-conscious agents of their own life and liberation" through transformative practices;[25] in essence, an Afrocentric practice of kriya yoga.

In 1966 Karenga created Kwanzaa, a seven-day Afrocentric observance for the worldwide Black community's "cultural recovery and reconstruction."[26] Traditionally observed the last week of the calendar year (December 26th through January 1st), with each day representing a specific value principle for reflection and contemplation, the Seven Nguzo Saba (seven principles) are rooted in ancient African spiritual and ethical principles as guidance for Blacks worldwide, and African Americans particularly, as a means of reinforcing communitarian values that will strengthen Black families, Black communities, and Black culture.

In his 2022 Annual Founder's Kwanzaa Message, Karenga writes:

> Kwanzaa was and is also an instrument of freedom, a means of cultivating liberated and liberating consciousness, returning us to our history and culture, and building and strengthening our families and communities in culturally-grounded ways that are good and transformative and cause us to flourish and come into the fullness of ourselves as African persons and peoples. Indeed, it opens up horizons of sensitivities, thoughts, possibilities and practices essential to reimagining and successfully struggling to bring into being a new history, hope and world for African peoples and humankind as a whole.[27]

The Yoga Sutras of Patanjali teach us that the practice of yoga will guide us toward the human goal of knowing the true self or self-realization. In order to meet this lifelong goal, we must first begin to identify the obstacles that keep us from enjoying the path of this life journey and this is due to our own spiritual ignorance (*avidya*) and thus our lack of understanding of our true selves. African Americans embrace the concept of liberation as a means of self-realization and reaching higher consciousness that is grounded in Christian, Islamic, and ancient African practices; these practices are tangible aspects that align with the yogic principles. Encouraging Black Americans to embrace the practice of yoga through this lens would only strengthen their quest for a healthy lifestyle and further their goal of obtaining true liberation that can only begin with a study of the self (*svadhyaya*). Our sojourn as Blacks in

America, reliance on our faith, and spiritual practices are reminiscent of Sutra 2:1 "Accepting pain as help for purification, study, and surrender to the Supreme Being constitute yoga practice."[28]

— CHAPTER 8 —

Who "Owns" Yoga?

With the popularity of yoga growing exponentially in the United States and around the world, many are exercising the freedom to usurp yoga in their own style and manner, and packaging such under unique brands that basically provide the same thing: yoga. However, is this prevailing practice yoga?

In 2011 Bikram Choudhry, the founder of Bikram yoga, attempted a lawsuit against an independent yoga studio founded by one of his former students. Choudhry claimed that the studio was offering yoga sequences formatted and based on the 26 yoga postures that constituted "Bikram" yoga, in violation of his self-claimed copyright on this yoga sequence. Choudhry not only lost his argument, but the United States Copyright Office also issued a policy clarification in the Federal Registry on the use and practices of yoga being universal and uncopyrightable. "The Copyright Office takes the position that a selection, coordination, or arrangement of functional physical movements such as sports movements, exercises, [or the selected arrangement of yoga poses], and other ordinary motor activities alone do not represent the type of authorship intended to be protected under the copyright law as a choreographic work."[1]

With the popularity of yoga growing exponentially in the United States and around the world, many are exercising the freedom to usurp yoga in their own style and manner, and packaging such under unique brands that basically provide the same thing: yoga. However, is this prevailing practice *yoga*?

Yoga has a 6000+ year history of practice with foundations in India and South Asia. Yoga philosophy was infused throughout Indian culture and religious practice yet, "as a function of colonialism (which began in

India around 1100 CE) these yoga practices were separated from Yoga the philosophy," writes Shyam Ranganathan, PhD, a professor of Indian philosophy in Toronto, Canada. "Once things called yoga are disconnected from Yoga, they can be used for various colonizing ends. Add to this branding, and you get a diversity of styles of yoga: all marketing."[2]

Scholars and practitioners of yoga in the West are contemplating the viewpoints on the cultural appropriation of yoga. Cultural appropriation is not a new concept. The United States is considered the "melting pot" of the world with the creed of the Statue of Liberty—America's beacon of freedom—beseeching the nations to "Give me your tired, your poor, your huddled masses yearning to breathe free, the wretched refuse of your teeming shore, send these the homeless, tempest-tossed to me, I lift my lamp beside the golden door!"[3] The huddling of masses from around the world pouring into one "pot" (nation) assures that a multitude of rituals, beliefs, and cultures are vying for voice and legitimacy of the people who carry these legacies.

"The practice of repurposing culture is as old as culture itself," notes Lauren Michele Jackson, author of *White Negroes: When Cornrows Were in Vogue...and Other Thoughts on Cultural Appropriation*, "and America has been making other cultures appropriate to its amusement and ambitions since the very beginning."[4] Jackson acknowledges that cultural appropriation is inevitable in a multi-cultural and multi-racial society and that this inevitability adds a richness to the society as a whole. However, by definition, cultural appropriation is deliberately taking or using any aspect of a culture that is not one's own and, when doing so, the practice is not properly acknowledged and/or practiced in a manner that shows true understanding of that culture. Cultural appropriation in this context is a detriment to societies that follow such practices because it establishes a power dynamic that allows the "appropriator" to use another's culture on their own terms, diminishing the value of the culture or race that is appropriated.[5]

Historically, this is especially true for African American culture. Since the time of enslavement, African and Black cultural appropriation practices have become a mainstay for burgeoning American society. "White people are not penalized for flaunting black culture—they are rewarded for doing so, financially, artistically, socially, and intellectually."[6] African American culinary cuisine, music, dance, and art cultures have all received adaptations within white society that took such cultural claims as their own. The minstrel shows of the past where white performers appeared in black face and vernacular, has segued to contemporary pop stars racializing their physical features by enlarging their lips, breasts, and bottoms to appropriate their view of white-styled Black women.[7]

For South Asians of India who embrace a yoga lifestyle, the Western cultural appropriation of the practice is experienced as a violation of their language, culture, and spiritual customs. Just as indigenous spiritual artifacts were stolen from Africa during the slave trade and sold as ornaments for the wealthy to display as exotic treasures (this continues today), South Asians experience the same indignities to their heritage. Americans displaying Hindu deities inappropriately on the floors or walls within their commercial yoga studios, inking tattoos of Sanskrit vows such as om/aum and namaste as body decoration, and misusing the concept of yoga philosophy as solely a performance of yoga postures (asanas) is offensive to a culture that considers yoga a sacred practice. "As yoga teachers and business owners, we have to question this," writes Arundhati Baitmangalkar, a yoga teacher of South Asian descent. "What have we done with yoga that has made it so alienating that individuals from the very culture that yoga originated in do not feel safe, respected, and accepted?"[8]

Perhaps this misappropriation of yoga culture is due to the naivety of Western practitioners or their misunderstanding of how yoga came to be present in the Western hemisphere in the first place. Unpacking the history of yoga's emergence in the United States, we find a much different aim and purpose from those who initiated this spiritual path in the West.

CHAPTER 9

The Gift of Yoga— East Meets West

The early yogis believed their sojourn in America was divinely guided and that they were sent to the far Western hemisphere to explain the deeper meaning of the reality of the Supreme Being and God consciousness in mankind.

As one of the newest nations on the scene in the 19th and 20th centuries, the United States represented the Wild West in everything good, bad, or decadent in human development. The growing elite class of European Americans were influenced by the philosophers and intellectual minds of the time, such as Sigmund Freud and Carl Jung, exploring ideas on the reality of God and mankind's role in perfectionism. The liberalism of philosophic thought amongst the elite offered an avenue for Indian yogis to inform a new spiritual aspect to traditional religious thought and practices in the United States.

Foundations of yoga practices in the West

The earliest gurus of yoga who came to teach in America represented their lineages of Indian yoga philosophy. In yoga terminology, "lineage refers to the historical succession of knowledge passed from teacher to teacher. With the foundation of lineage, a disciple of yoga gains insight not only from his/her own teacher, but from all the teachers that came before."[1]

The common experience amongst these gurus is that all were sent by their own master gurus to the West to share the universality of yoga as a spiritual path that transcends religions. These early gurus also changed the culture of yoga discipleship. Yoga was historically taught master/teacher to disciple/pupil, but the gurus who transformed yoga in the United States often taught large groups of students as early forms of yoga teacher training. A few gurus, such as Swami Paramahansa Yogananda and Swami Satchidananda Saraswati, did eventually offer discipleship through a contemporary monastic initiation.

1893	1920	1956	1960–1969
Swami Vivekananda	Paramahansa Yogananda	B.K.S. Iyengar	Satchidananda Saraswati T.K.V. Desikachar Sri K. Pattabhi Jois Amrit Desai Harbhajan Singh Khalsa

FIGURE 9.1 TIMELINE OF YOGA LINEAGE IN AMERICA

These early yogis believed that their sojourn in America was divinely guided and that they were sent to the far Western hemisphere to explain the deeper meaning of the reality of the Supreme Being and God consciousness in mankind. These initial introductions of yoga to the West were not as a physical practice such as asana or hatha yoga per se, however they provided insight to spirituality as a focus of the yogic principles of dharana (direct concentration of the mind), dhyana (meditation), pranayama (breathing), and samadhi (spiritual ecstasy or bliss).

Swami Vivekananda: jnana yoga

The earliest recorded Indian thought philosopher to visit and teach in America was Swami Vivekananda. Vivekananda was a practicing Hindu and monastic disciple of Sri Ramakrishna's spiritual lineage, who taught jnana yoga, a traditional path of the Vedanta[2] known as nondualism: "the wisdom associated with discerning the Real from the unreal or illusory."[3] In 1893, at the age of 30, Vivekananda attended the World Parliament of Religions in Chicago, Illinois. America was thus introduced to the teachings of the Bhagavad Gita through his keynote speech, which included the Hindu precept that all religions are from one source. "Through his teachings on the four yogas [karma, bhakti, jnana, and raja], the harmony of religions, divinity of the soul, and serving humanity as God, Vivekananda gave spiritual aspirants paths to that realization."[4]

One year later, in 1894, Vivekananda would establish a formal foundation for Hindu thought and practice in the United States as the Vedanta Society of New York. The Vedanta Society remains active today with 15 centers in the United States as well as practicing societies in India and around the world.

Swami Yogananda: kriya yoga

Swami Paramahansa Yogananda's sojourn in the United States would set the foundation for yoga as a formal institution in the West. Considered the "Father of Yoga in the West," his ministry provided an avenue for exploring the deeper underlying "principles of truth that are common foundations of all religious practices."[5] Yogananda's teachings exemplified the "original Christianity of Jesus Christ and the original Yoga of the Bhagavan Krishna: Krishna [being] the divine exemplar of yoga in the East; Christ [being] chosen by God as the exemplar of God-union for the West."[6]

Sent to the United States by his guru lineage, Yogananda's primary message was the unity of all religions and individual development of the personal relationship with the Divine. Through kriya yoga, Yogananda explained that spirituality is a science, unlike religions that profess a specific creed or dogma. The goal of the spiritual messages of all religions is acknowledging the Supreme Being within oneself. The practice of self-realization, kriya yoga, provides a formalized technique of meditation that allows the practitioners the means for achieving enlightenment by awakening the internal cosmic force within the self.

Achieving spiritual enlightenment and calling from an early age, Yogananda was a disciple of Sri Yukteswar Giri, a monastic who believed to have received the divine knowledge of kriya yoga from the Supreme Being through his own guru lineage (Swami Order of Shankaracharya).

In 1920, Yogananda visited and taught in Boston, Massachusetts, and gave his first formal lecture in America to the Congress of Religious Liberals. Migrating to Los Angeles in 1925, Yogananda founded the first Self-Realization Fellowship Society (SRF). During his 32 years living and teaching throughout the United States and the world, Yogananda taught millions of people and established SRF societies including a monastic order for serious discipleship throughout the major cities of America.

As a brown-skinned Indian, Yogananda would experience racism that was prevalent in the United States during that time, especially in the South. During a visit to Washington, DC that afforded speaking engagements with members of the United States Congress and then President Calvin Coolidge, Yogananda learned of the segregation laws (Jim Crow) that restricted African Americans from attending his lectures. Steadfast in his belief in the universal message of kriya yoga, Yogananda made efforts to establish SRF societies for African Americans and in 1927 formed the first Afro-American Yogoda Association in Washington, DC.[7]

Yogananda's Self-Realization Fellowship and Yogoda Satsanga Society organizations continue today following his aim "to point out the one divine highway to which all paths of true religious beliefs eventually lead: the highway of daily scientific, devotional meditation on God."[8]

Swami Satchidananda: integral yoga

The teachings of integral yoga were introduced in the United States by Swami Satchidananda Saraswati, a disciple of Swami Sivananda Saraswati, a Hindu philosopher and yogi. Satchidananda's influence and impact on yoga in the 20th century expanded both the interfaith spirituality and the integrative healthcare movements. In 1969 Satchidananda came into prominence as a keynote speaker at the Woodstock Music venue where he acknowledged to the congregate festival participants that as America leads the world in materialism, in the spirit of Woodstock, it now needs to lead the world in spirituality. He later counseled with multiple celebrities including musicians George Harrison of the Beatles, jazz composer Alice Coltrane, and singer-songwriter Carole King.

Pressing that integral yoga is a lifestyle, Satchidananda supported scientific research on the use of yoga therapy in integrative health modalities and worked with Dean Ornish, a medical researcher from Harvard University who later became a follower and practitioner of integral yoga. Satchidananda further supported the teachings of yoga as therapy in both drug rehabilitation centers and prisons in New York and Virginia.

Satchidananda was a founding member of the Yoga Alliance and developed one of the first yoga teaching training certification programs in the United States. The Integral Yoga Institute includes the first yoga magazine and publishing company for the transliterations of important yoga texts, the Bhagavad Gita and the Yoga Sutras of Patanjali.

In the spirit of other Indian yogis who were sent to the West to spread the teachings of Eastern spirituality, Satchidananda counseled with religious and spiritual teachers of all faiths. In 1986 he dedicated the Light of Truth Universal Shrine (LOTUS) at Integral Yoga's ashram in Virginia, Yogaville. The shrine includes altars for various faith traditions from around the world. In 2014 a LOTUS shrine was built in India.

Swami Krishnamacharya: therapeutic hatha yoga

Although the majority of the earlier Indian yoga gurus brought a universal spiritual message and method of enlightenment to the West, the work of the disciples of Tirumalai Krishnamacharya emphasized the physical therapeutic aspects of the yoga practice, hatha yoga.

Tirumalai Krishnamacharya was a yoga teacher and healer within the Indian medical science of ayurveda who lived and worked for one whole century (1888–1999). With the privilege of working for the King of Mysore in the 1930s, he mastered yoga philosophy and created forms of yoga practices that aligned physical movements with the breath (vinyasa). Considered the architect of viniyoga, Krishnamacharya incorporated his hatha yoga style of alignment with the practices of ayurveda where the healing modalities were individualized for his clients or patients.

The disciples of Krishnamacharya include three prominent Indian yogis who shared his teachings in America. Krishnamacharya's son, **Tirumalai Krishnamacharya Venkata Desikachar** (T.K.V. Desikachar), further developed the practices of viniyoga as a holistic healing art. T.K.V. Desikachar carried the legacy of his father to teach yoga philosophy as an individualized approach for all people regardless of their body type, age, health status, or cultural background. He did not wish to be associated with a specific "style" of yoga, but rather taught yoga as a means to understanding one's individual lifestyle journey. Desikachar, like his father, taught yoga as an instrument for practitioners to develop an intimate relationship with Ultimate Reality. "Anyone who can breathe can do Yoga," Desikachar would say. "It is the practical means by which the ideals of an inspired life can be actualized."[9]

In 1976 Desikachar founded a yoga teacher training and research center: Krishnamacharya Yoga Mandiram in Madras, India. Desikachar's yoga therapy research included yoga practice for mental health conditions such as schizophrenia and depression, among other health modalities.

Sri K. Pattabhi Jois would meld his guru's teaching into a hatha yoga system he coined as "ashtanga" that includes the use of pranayama (breathing), bandhas (core muscular and energetic locks), drishti (visual focal points), and asanas practiced in a vinyasa style of flowing movements. Pattabhi Jois is recognized for presenting the *surya nam-askar* (sun salutation) as a focus of vinyasa practice.

Pattabhi Jois began his study of yoga under Krishnamacharya at age 14 in Mysore, India. Well educated, he would serve as a professor of philosophy and Sanskrit scholar for the Maharaja. Pattabhi Jois authored his manual of ashtanga yoga—*Yoga Mala*—that outlines his ethical principles and philosophy of ashtanga yoga. In his ashtanga yoga system, students primarily practice the physical postures (asanas) as a vinyasa (flow) before learning other aspects of the eight limbs of yoga as originally codified by Patanjali.

Bellur Krishnamachar Sundararaja Iyengar (B.K.S. Iyengar) is the founder of Iyengar yoga: a hatha yoga style practice that revolutionized the use of props and physical adjustments in yoga. His seminal book, *Light on Yoga*, is considered "The bible of modern yoga," an encyclopedia of yoga postures and hatha yoga sequences to support overall health and chronic diseases.[10] Iyengar yoga also follows the tenets of Patanjali's eight limbs of yoga (ashtanga), and encourages a daily routine of hatha yoga as "the young, the old, the extremely aged, even the sick and the firm obtain perfection in Yoga by constant practice."[11]

B.K.S. Iyengar first visited the United States in 1956 at the invitation of the violin maestro Yehudi Menuhin. He was the first to teach hatha yoga to large groups of students. Iyengar's hatha yoga is grounded on the principles of physical alignment as the means of establishing good physical health and vitality. B.K.S. Iyengar was considered a "house holder" having married and sired children who would further their father's work through the Ramamani Iyengar Memorial Yoga Institute (RIMYI) in Pune, India. B.K.S. Iyengar's daughter, Geeta Iyengar, especially supported yoga practices for women's health. His son Prashant Iyengar continues the work of his father today as the leader of RIMYI.

The growing popularity of restorative yoga is greatly influenced by the practice and work of Judith Lasater, who studied under B.K.S. Iyengar at RIMYI. Lasater's publication *Relax and Renew: Restful Yoga for Stressful Times* highlights the therapeutic benefits of a hatha yoga and pranayama practice.[12]

Amrit Desai: Kripalu yoga

Kripalu yoga is named for Yogacharya Swami Kripalvananda, an Indian philosopher, ayurvedic practitioner, and yoga master. Kripalvananda's student, Amrit Desai, who introduced Kripalu yoga in the United States, met his guru in India at the age of 15. After studying for decades with Kripalvananda, Amrit Desai began teaching yoga in Philadelphia, Pennsylvania, where he was attending art school. Returning to India in 1966, Amrit Desai was initiated into kundalini yoga by his guru. He returned to the United States with his guru's blessing and founded a residential yoga center in Pennsylvania. This work would forge the Kripalu Healing Arts Institute dedicated to holistic health and healing and the development of formalized yoga, yoga therapy, and ayurveda training for Western practitioners. The Kripalu Institute's "history parallels the evolution of yoga in America, which progresses from an exclusive reliance on Eastern tradition, teachers, and cultural forms, to the development of Western teachers steeped in the [yoga] tradition."[13]

In 2023, at the age of 90, Gurudev Shri Amritji continues to teach and lead yoga at the Amrit Yoga Institute in Florida, and his "lineage of light" legacy is furthered through his daughter Kamini Desai who carries the title of Yogeshwari (woman of yoga mastery) "for her keen ability to bring ancient illumination to genuine challenges of the human spirit."[14]

Yogi Bhajan: kundalini yoga

A distinctive style of yoga was introduced to America by Harbhajan Singh Khalsa, a practitioner of the Sikh religious tradition. Yogi Bhajan cultivated a practice of kundalini yoga, a systematic practice for personal enlightenment that includes kriyas (actions), meditation, chanting, asana, and yoga philosophy to assist the practitioner in accessing their own inner spiritual light as a means to healing and holiness.

Through the Sikh tradition, "Yogi Bhajan was given the unique ministerial position of Siri Singh Sahib of Sikh Dharma (Chief Religious and Administrative Authority) of the Western Hemisphere."[15] With over 300 kundalini centers in 35 countries, Bhajan's missionary work would inspire both Sikhs and non-Sikhs worldwide seeking spiritual enlightenment.

Bhajan was born in Pakistan. In his youth he studied kundalini under the enlightened teacher Sant Hazara Singh, who blessed Bhajan as a master of kundalini at the age of 16. In 1947 Bhajan and members of his village immigrated to India during a war that led to the partitioning of Pakistan from India. A highly educated man, he later traveled to the West, first arriving in Canada in 1968 to teach yoga at Toronto University before migrating to Los Angeles, California, where he formally established the kundalini yoga community.

Bhajan emphasized the science of kundalini as an alternative method of healing and achieving bliss states of ecstasy that the American baby boomer generation of the 1960s were striving to find within the prevailing drug culture of the time. Based on his first principle of "Happiness is a birthright," Bhajan founded the 3HO (Healthy, Happy, and Holy Organization) in 1969. 3HO would evolve to further his missionary work that included the development of health-related products and services with followers incorporating their own professional skills as chiropractors, acupuncturists, and nutritionists within the yogic principles of healing. In 1994 3HO became a member of the United Nations as a non-governmental organization (NGO) "representing women's issues, promoting human rights and providing education in alternative systems of medicine."[16]

Post lineage contemporary practices of yoga in the West

As the popularity of yoga grew in the United States, a multitude of yoga styles began to emerge. These contemporary yoga styles were established by Westerners outside of the traditional Indian yoga lineages, although some were influenced by the early Indian yoga masters.

The primary style for American yoga is based on the somatic practice of asana (hatha yoga). Initially, the appeal of these new ways of teaching and practicing yoga was primarily to young, affluent European American women, and would later prove for some of these founders of the American yoga movement to be divided by ethical scandals. The appropriation of Indian yoga culture also became a focus of debate for these new forms of yoga due to alleged misuse of Indian philosophical ideals, Sanskrit, and deity worship outside the context of Indian culture.

Because of this, national and international yoga-based organizations adopted codes and conduct and ethical standards for their members and to assure that the public seeking yoga practices are in safe and respectful spaces. Yoga Alliance (YA), the largest registry and non-profit organization representing the yoga community both nationally and internationally, adopted an ethical commitment that unifies "members around shared principles and to foster safe and respectful guidelines for the profession of yoga teaching."[17] YA's ethical commitment consists of three requirements: (1) a code of conduct that defines the proper behavior of yoga teachers with their students, including consent to touch and honesty in communication; (2) a scope of practice that describes the role of yoga teachers and defines the core competencies needed to provide a yoga teaching practice; and (3) responsibility to equity in yoga that defines YA's commitment to assuring members and the public are treated equitably within yoga spaces.

Here are brief descriptions of the more popular yoga styles practiced in America in alphabetical order:

Anusara School of Hatha Yoga Founded by John Friend in 1997, anusara is a hatha yoga practice that focuses on the qualities of the heart (practicing yoga with the right attitude) and the universal principles of alignment that have become its trademark. Friend's hatha yoga practice was influenced by Krishnamacharya's disciples Pattabhi Jois and B.K.S. Iyengar.

Anusara's universal principles of alignment prescribe creative anatomical language such as the use of "muscular energy" to describe the engagement of muscles to support skeletal structure (i.e., "hug the muscles to the bones"); "inner and outer spirals" to describe internal and external rotations of the joints; and "organic energy" that describes the dynamic movement of energy from the body's inner core to the peripheral extremities.

Baptiste Institute Founded by Baron Baptiste, Baptiste yoga is a power flow (vinyasa) style that includes 53 postures (asanas) that are linked in a practice that focuses on concentration of drishti (focused gaze) *ujjayi* (breath), bandhas (foundation), and tapas (heat). Baron Baptiste grew up in a yoga tradition, his parents being students of B.K.S. Iyengar and his disciple, Indra Devi. The Baptistes were early pioneers of the American yoga movement, opening yoga schools in San Francisco in the early 1950s.

The influence of the Iyengar style of hatha yoga on the Baptiste Institute is best summarized in Baron Baptiste's explanation for the purpose of his form of yoga, "It is my mission to make yoga accessible to anyone, from any background, who is looking for total physical, mental, and emotional transformation."[18]

Bikram Yoga Bikram Choudhury developed a version of vinyasa (flow) yoga that includes 26 standard postures (asanas) that are practiced in studios heated at 104 degrees Fahrenheit (40 degrees Celsius). Bikram Choudhury credits the influence of his yoga style to Bishnu Charan

Ghosh, an Indian bodybuilder and hatha yogi who taught hatha yoga as exercise. B.C. Ghosh is the younger brother of Paramahansa Yogananda.

Often called "hot yoga," to simulate India's environmental climate, Bikram style follows a formal script of teaching the specific 26 yoga postures (asanas) and includes rigorous pranayama practice known as "breath of fire" (*kapalabhati*).

Yin Yoga Yin yoga is an adaptation of hatha yoga where specific yoga postures (asanas) are held passively for longer periods of time, yet differs from restorative yoga in that the postures held are meant to present both physical and mindful challenges, and not stimulate relaxation. Popularized by Paul Grilley and his student Sarah Powers, yin yoga is based on the Daoist practice of Chi Kung. Grilley adapted the slower paced yin practice as a balance to the more popular "yang-style" yoga practices of ashtanga-power and vinyasa flow classes. Powers is credited in naming yin yoga as a style of yoga and included the alignment of the traditional Chinese medicine (TCM) energetic meridian channels within the yin yoga system to explain the physiological and energetic benefits of a yin yoga practice.

The three main principles of yin yoga practice are: (1) ease into the shape of the posture (asana) that can be held and tolerated for a specific period of time; (2) find a point of stillness so that joints can be nourished, and mind can become calm; and (3) hold the posture long enough for the specific meridian channel to be nourished, similar to the experience of acupuncture.[19]

YogaSkills school of kemetic yoga As summarized in Chapter 3, "Kemetic yoga refers to an entire spiritual system of self-development created by the sages of ancient Egypt. It is a worldview that recognizes the nature of reality and our place in the universe."[20]

Founded by Master Yirser Ra Hotep, YogaSkills kemetic yoga is based on the scientific research of Egyptian cosmology he conducted along with his teacher Dr. Asar Hapi in the 1970s. Their research documents that "yoga in all its forms was practiced in Egypt earlier than anywhere else in history,"[21] reasoning that yoga's foundation is rooted in African culture. Egypt, as the seat of civilization, gave birth to spiritual philosophies that influenced many faith traditions within the monotheistic and polytheistic systems and cosmologies. Scholars of kemetic yoga "note that the major forms of Indian yoga can be found in ancient Egyptian scriptures, inscribed in papyrus and on temple walls as well as steles, statues, obelisks and other sources."[22]

Unlike contemporary forms of Indian-styled yoga practiced in the United States, kemetic yoga is practiced at a slower pace with a focus on breath (prana), meditation, and opening of the energy centers (chakras) of the body.[23] The physical postures (asanas) of kemetic yoga form the shapes of ancient drawings and hieroglyphics depicting the Egyptian gods and goddesses. Similar to other forms of yoga, the main theme of Egyptian or kemetic yoga is self-realization: to realize that our "eternal souls come to earth to learn certain lessons and become purified."[24]

With over 8000 teachers trained worldwide, kemetic yoga provides an Afrocentric outlet for Black people seeking to know more about their own culture through a spiritual practice that parallels the yogic principles of traditional Indian yoga.

CHAPTER 10

The Universality of Yoga

As a student-teacher of yoga, we are facilitators of the practice, striving to understand our own human nature as a means of encouraging those that practice with us to begin the journey toward understanding their unique human nature.

The view of yoga from the American lens is a kaleidoscope of interpretations on a theme that, in best practice, maintains yoga's philosophic foundations of origin. The universal appeal of yoga is the basis of its path as a journey toward spiritual enlightenment and its adaptability within the various cultural nuances that humankind has evolved over time. However, when aspects of yoga, or any faith tradition, are extracted in a vacuum that disavows its genesis, the essence of the tradition is lost and rendered meaningless.

To successfully share a practice of yoga in the Black community, the genuine essence of the message must be clearly stated. The African American community has historically been short-changed by most of the health-promoting and lifestyle opportunities offered in America. Health promotions marketed to African Americans are highly biased and primarily for pharmaceutical remedies. For example, televised commercials that advertised diabetic medications for a disease that ranks highest amongst Black people depicted a sedentary family image of Black folk sitting around playing card games while eating high fat foods. Contrast this with other pharmaceutical commercials marketed toward the dominant culture, featuring Caucasian folks striving to be physically fit by biking, hiking, or practicing yoga on the beach.

Black civil rights activist Fanny Lou Hamer declared for herself and the Black community that we are "sick and tired of being sick and tired."[1] Standing on a lineage of African Americans whose backs were beaten and broken for desiring to be treated equitably, Fanny Lou Hamer, a symbol of resilience for Black people because of her activism, carried a legacy of physical, mental, and emotional trauma that proved to be detrimental for her own life and one that continues to resonate in the community she vowed to serve.

To be genuine in sharing a practice of yoga in the Black community, a yoga teacher must embrace the attributes of the "3 Cs": character, courage, and compassion for self and the community.

Character As yoga teachers, we are first and foremost students. Jesus reminds his disciples that to reach the kingdom of heaven one must embrace the humble state of a child.[2] The spirit of a child is one of curiosity and wonder for the unknown. The first question that most young children learn to speak and ask is "Why?"

No one can teach what one does not know. The standard 200-hour yoga teacher training program in the United States provides an elementary and cursory overview of the practice of yoga, and this is if the training program has aligned their curriculum with the core competencies standards outlined by the Yoga Alliance.[3] Yoga teachers must wholeheartedly embrace the niyama of *svadhyaya*: a study of the self and the Self (Supreme Being/Ultimate Reality/God Consciousness). As a student-teacher of yoga, we are facilitators of the practice, striving to understand our own human nature as a means of encouraging those that practice with us to begin the journey toward understanding their unique human nature. *Svadhyaya* is "lifelong learning." This is the first commitment to becoming a practitioner of yoga and a yoga teacher.

Courage As yoga teachers we must have the courage to admit our limitations and stay in our lane of knowledge and understanding. We must put our egos aside when challenges arise and consider these new opportunities to learn more about ourselves, the situation at hand, and life in general. Teaching yoga in the Black community requires a thorough knowledge of the impact of systematic racism, the disproportionate health disparities and other environmental challenges, such as those outlined in Part II, that are impacting our community. In today's climate, no one, especially Black people, is entering a yoga class completely healthy and whole. With a knowledge of our own selves (abilities and limitations) we yoga teachers are better equipped to hold space for yoga students who potentially feel vulnerable due to a history of ill treatment, ridiculing, microaggressions, or dismissiveness by others regarding our thoughts, feelings, and experiences.

"When yoga teachers, educators, and therapists lack critical awareness of race and racism, and have not adequately dealt with their own racial hang-ups," teaches Gail Parker, author of *Restorative Yoga for Ethnic and Race-Based Stress and Trauma*, "...and when they are uncomfortable and unprepared to deal with issues of race as they come up, they become part of the problem."[4]

Granted, it is not necessary to become confrontational or apologetic. However, the truth of the impact of daily living in a racist society cannot be underestimated or rationalized. Black folk need to begin to heal from the inside out. Yoga is a peaceful path that may support this journey when applied within the systematic spiritual science that Patanjali intended as an eight-limbed path to enlightenment. Beyond the intellectual discussions, yoga teachers are a living example of the practical application of the ashtanga eight limbs. To claim the attribute of "yogi/yogini" is to embody the practice.

Compassion for community In 2020 the *New York Times* published an article entitled "Black yoga collectives aim to make space for healing."[5] The article features a Black woman, the primary caregiver of her special needs daughter and father, whose story unfolds as she loses her only son in a senseless murder. Unfortunately, this narrative is not an unfamiliar experience for Blacks living in America today. However, this story shares the value of yoga and meditation as a coping strategy toward healing grief and loss. Beverly Grant, who is featured in the article, would grow in her yoga practice and begin teaching at Denver, Colorado's Satya Yoga Cooperative to "help individuals better process trauma and grief before it shows up in their bodies as mental health conditions and chronic diseases."[6] Recognizing that she is not alone, Ms. Grant learned the value of sharing her own healing journey and practice within her community.

First and foremost, the Black community needs our compassion. This is patiently empathizing with a traumatized group of people who do not wish to be patronized, but to at least be heard, if not understood. Everyone's desire is to heal. Yoga as a way of life is a way of love. Love of self and others. The two foundational building blocks of ashtanga—yama and niyama—provide us with tools to learn how to love oneself and how to love others. As yoga teachers, we begin sharing the journey of yoga by learning a respect for life that is in short supply for Blacks in American society.

Applying the yogic principles in a teaching practice

Yoga is a culturally responsive practice that may be adapted to harmonize with various racial, ethnic, and cultural groups' needs. Within the African American cultural context, the principles of humanity that resonate across our religious and spiritual belief systems are paths to the one truth. Table 10.1 offers a harmonizing of principles and practices as a means to a yoga practice within the Black community.

Table 10.1

Yogic principles	Christianity	Kwanzaa Nguzo Saba	Islam
Yama	Golden rule (Matthew 7:12)	Ujima/Self-determination Ujamaa/Collective work & responsibility	Charity/Zakat (Surah 4:36)
Niyama	Beatitudes (Matthew 5:3–12)	Kujichagulia/Cooperative economics	Pilgrimage/Hajj (Surah 2:197)
Asana	Body as temple (1 Corinthians 6:19–20)	Nia/Purpose	
Pranayama	Breath of spirit (Genesis 2:7)	Umoja	Belief in Allah/Muslim (Surah 2:136)
Pratyahara	Self-denial (Ephesians 4:22–24)	Kuumba/Creativity	Fasting/Siyam (Surah 2:183)
Dharana	Prayer (Philippians 4:6–7)	Imani/Faith	Prayer/Salat (Surah 29:45)
Dhyana	Wisdom of stillness (Psalm 46:10)		
Samadhi	God in the midst of you (Luke 17:20–21)		Faith/Islam (Surah 42:52–53)

Glossary of terms: religious and spiritual belief systems used in Table 10.1

Yogic principles[7]

The eight limbs of yoga are: yama (abstinence), niyama (observance), asana (posture), pranayama (breath control), pratyahara (sense withdrawal), dharana (concentration), dhyana (meditation), and samadhi (bliss) (Sutra 2:29).

Patanjali's ashtanga eight limbs of yoga system begins with the aspirant or seeker considering their relationship with others as well as their understanding of self. Yama and niyama follow the principle of the "Golden Rule," do unto others as one would do unto self.

Yama (Sutra 2.30) Follow the principle of abstinence. Seekers abstain from any interactions with others that would prove harmful to the relationship including abstaining from all forms of violence—physical or emotional (*ahimsa*), speaking the truth regardless of the circumstance (*satya*), honoring the gifts of others by not coveting what is not one's own (*asteya*), being patient and empathetic (*bramacharya*), and valuing others' gifts and talents in the absence of envy or jealousy (*aparigraha*).

Niyama (Sutra 2.32) Follow the principle of introspection or observance. Seekers' inner observances are quiet reflections on one's purity of heart (*saucha*), contentment of mind (*santosha*), acceptance of one's own limitations as potential areas of growth (*tapas*), and through the commitment to cultivate one's journey as lifelong learners (*svadhyaya*), surrender to the source of life by worshiping God (*ishvara pranidhana*).

As the seeker continues their inner work of self-restraint (yama) and introspection (niyama), the practice of ashtanga graduates to active physical preparations to master the fluctuations of the mind that lead to the distractions that hinder our goal of finding the joy that life promises.

Asana (Sutra 2:46) The health and vitality of our physical body supports the preparation for the deeper mental and spiritual practices of yoga. The goal of the asana practice is the development of a steady comfortable posture for meditation. An undisciplined body will not ease the mind. Through the asana practice the seeker learns to adjust to the sensations that our bodies experience as they flow through the daily actions of life and learns to observe how these sensations influence our thoughts.

Pranayama (Sutra 2:49) The subtle blessing of the breath is the source of life that most of us take for granted. The absence of breath is death. Pranayama is a practice that honors the breath as the source of life. The seeker strives to move in harmony with the breath, enjoying the various rhythmic patterns that, when mastered, elevate mood, stimulate relaxation, and assure a calm presence.

Pratyahara (Sutra 2:504) Human beings are blessed with five basic senses: sight, hearing, touch, smell, and taste. Our sense perception shapes our view of the world and how we interact with it. Through the practice of pratyahara, secession from how we sense the world moves us away from our biases, and we begin a practice of viewing life with objectivity.

Dharana (Sutra 3:1) The practice of dharana is to the mind as the practice of asana is to the physical body. The seeker's ability to concentrate opens the channels for meditation by strengthening their ability to focus the fluctuations of thoughts that distract us from the object of meditation.

Dhyana (Sutra 3:3) The evolution of humanity is aided by our ability to activate our sixth sense, intuition. Dhyana, the practice of meditation, moves the seeker from striving to control life from the limited view and comfort of our perspective, to observing life as it unfolds.

Samadhi (Sutra 1:17) The pleasure of samadhi is in its practical application. Samadhi is the reward of joy we experience from our progression through the eight limbs. The bliss of feeling the reality of God Consciousness each time we evolve in our understanding of life's lessons is the subtle gaining of wisdom that makes us a practicing yogi/yogini.

Christianity[8]

The Christian faith is simple but its numerous interpretations can be complex. The interpretations of the faith are as varietal as Mother Nature's botanicals. The debate over whether Christians can or cannot practice yoga is tied to a belief that every action (such as meditation or asana) may be devotional and thus a deviation from one's faith. A practice of discernment would benefit this discussion. Meditation is a tenet of Christianity when the believer's meditation practice is on the word of God. Our bodies and spirits are the gifts of God and therefore should be honored with proper care, such as a movement through a practice of asana. (3 John 1:2) Beloved, I pray that all may go well with you and you may be in good health, as it goes well with your soul.

Many faiths believe that God created us all in His image and like-ness—His nature, and there are many paths taken to discover truth. Converging paths are harmonized by understanding their core principles and practices as humanity is a practice of yoga. Employing principles and practices that support one faith is not necessarily a construct of religion. "Any form of Christian yoga—is not a religion," writes Brooke Boon, author of *Holy Yoga*. "Rather, it is a practice of bodily alignment, mindful breathing, and purposeful reliance on God."[9]

The following Biblical scriptures offer a contemplative practice for self and community care.

Golden Rule (Matthew 7:12) So whatever you wish that others would do to you, do also to them, for this is the Law and the Prophets.

Beatitudes (Matthew 5:3–12) Blessed are the poor in spirit, for theirs is the kingdom of heaven. Blessed are those who mourn, for they shall be comforted. Blessed are the meek, for they shall inherit the earth. Blessed are those who hunger and thirst for righteousness, for they shall be satisfied. Blessed are the merciful, for they shall receive mercy. Blessed are the pure in heart, for they shall see God. Blessed are they who are persecuted for righteousness' sake, for theirs is the kingdom of heaven. Blessed are you when others revile you and persecute you, and utter all kinds of evil against you falsely on my account. Rejoice and be glad, for your reward is great in heaven, for so they persecuted the prophets who were before you.

Body as temple (1 Corinthians 6:19–20) Or, do you not know that your body is a temple of the Holy Spirit within you, whom you have from God? You are not your own, for you were bought with a price. So glorify God in your body.

Breath of Spirit (Genesis 2:7) Then the Lord God formed man of the dust of the ground, and breathed into his nostrils the breath of life; and man became a living creature.

Self-denial (Ephesians 4:22–24) To put off your old self, which belongs to your former manner of life and is corrupt through deceitful desires, and to be renewed in the spirit of your minds, and to put on the new self, created after the likeness of God in true righteousness and holiness.

Prayer (Philippians 4:6–7) Do not be anxious about anything, but in everything by prayer and supplication with thanksgiving let your requests be known to God. And the peace of God, which surpasses all understanding, will guard your hearts and your minds in Christ Jesus.

Wisdom of stillness (Psalm 46:10) Be still, and know that I am God: I will be exalted among the nations, I will be exalted in the earth!

God in the midst of you (Luke 17:20–21) The kingdom of God is not coming in ways that can be observed, nor will they say "Look, here it is!" or "There!" for behold, the kingdom of God is in the midst of you.

Kwanzaa principles[10]

The application of the seven Nguzo Saba (seven principles) of Kwanzaa "is our duty, to know our past and honor it; to engage our present and improve it; and to imagine a whole new future and forge it in the most ethical, effective, and expansive ways."[11]

The seven principles of Kwanzaa are traditionally observed in seven consecutive days in the sequence listed below. The principles may also be practiced as monthly, quarterly, or annual observances to more fully explore the deep, rich meaning of each.

Umoja (unity) To strive for and maintain unity in the family, community, nation, and race.

Kujichagulia (self-determination) To define ourselves, name ourselves, create for ourselves, and speak for ourselves.

Ujima (collective work and responsibility) To build and maintain our community together, and make our brothers' and sisters' problems our problems, and to solve them together.

Ujamaa (cooperative economics) To build and maintain our stores, shops, and other businesses, and to profit from them together.

Nia (purpose) To make our collective vocation the building and developing of our community to restore our people to their traditional greatness.

Kuumba (creativity) To always do as much as we can, in the way we can, in order to leave our community more beautiful and beneficial than we inherited it.

Imani (faith) To believe with all our heart, in our people, our parents, our teachers, and our leaders and the righteousness and victory of our struggle.

Islam[12]

A beauty of Islam is that there is no compulsion in the religion (Surah 2:256). Wisdom is gained through the choices one makes in life; we are all responsible for the consequences of our actions. When one chooses to embrace the Islamic faith, the believer then commits to its pillars (living standards) that are designed to strengthen one's humanity as representatives of God on earth.

The following Quranic scriptures offer a contemplative practice for self and community care.

Belief in God/Muslim Acknowledging in all walks of life, reverence for the source of all life, the Supreme Being. (Surah 2:136) Say: We believe in Allah and (in) that which has been revealed to us, and (in) that which was revealed to Abraham, and Ishmael and Isaac and Jacob and the tribes, and (in) that which was given to Moses and Jesus, and (in) that which was given to the prophets from their Lord, we do not make any distinction between any of them and to Him do we submit.

Charity/Zakat As God has gifted us with all the wealth, faculties and powers that we possess, our action of benevolence is sharing what we have to assure the goodness of humanity. (Surah 4:36) Serve Allah and ascribe no partner to Him. Do good to your parents, to near of kin, to orphans, and to the needy, and to the neighbor who is of kin and to the neighbor who is a stranger, and to the companion by your side, and to the wayfarer, and to those whom your right hand possesses.

Fasting/Siyam Fasting is a spiritual discipline of abstinence: it strengthens our will power and purifies our hearts and minds. (Surah 2:183) O you who believe, fasting is prescribed for you, as it was prescribed for those before you, so that you may guard against evil.

Faith/Islam Faith is the commitment to obtaining the highest moral qualities of humanity established by God and requires active participation in living the divine attributes as the goal of one's life. (Surah 42:52–53) And thus did We reveal to thee an inspired Book by our command. Thou knewest not what the book was nor (what) Faith (was), but We made it a light, guiding thereby whom We please of our servants. And surely thou guidest to the right path—The path of Allah, to Whom belongs whatsoever is in the heavens and whatsoever is in the earth. Now surely to Allah do all affairs eventually come.

Pilgrimage/Hajj The faithful journey toward the Divine. (Surah 2:197) The months of the pilgrimage are well known, so whoever determines to perform pilgrimage therein there shall be no immodest speech, nor abusing, nor altercation in the pilgrimage. And whatever good you do, Allah knows it. And make provision for yourselves, the best provision being to keep one's duty. And keep your duty to Me, O men of understanding.

Prayer/Salat Prayer is our first duty in the onward progress of human development as prayer helps us to realize the Divine within the self and provides the humility needed to attain the highest degree of moral and spiritual perfection. (Surah 21:45) Recite that which has been revealed to thee of the Book and keep up prayer. Surely prayer keeps (one) away from indecency and evil; and certainly, the remembrance of Allah is the greatest (force). And Allah knows what you do.

— PART IV —

SHARING THE PRACTICE IN THE BLACK COMMUNITY

This section is about yoga as a practice of healing and should serve as a primer and a source of references as you begin your teaching journey, if further inquiry piques your interest, or you want to further the perspective of your current yoga practice. General introductory information is provided. The book addresses the proverbial tip of the iceberg. The path of inquiry is part of a beautiful lifelong endeavor. Healing is a personal journey and yoga facilitates that healing through the use of tools that practitioners can use throughout a lifetime, in many settings, and under numerous circumstances. So, consider this book to be a primer, a short introduction to get you started or restarted.

Yoga is a lifestyle practice that can be particularly beneficial as part of the efforts to improve health within the Black community. Medicine has progressed in controlling communicable diseases to a point where these diseases are no longer a substantial cause of death throughout the world.[1] Noncommunicable diseases (NCD) are now the major cause of death globally. Lifestyle is the major cause of NCDs. The four major disease groups that the World Health Organization says contribute to NCD deaths are cardiovascular disease, cancer, diabetes, and respiratory disease. Eighty percent of NCD deaths are attributed to these four disease groups. These four disease groups, among others, are prevalent in the Black community. In addition to tobacco and alcohol use, physical inactivity and unhealthy diet are major causes of these four disease groups. .

Chronic stress also impacts NCDs. In its 2014 *Stress in America* survey, the American Psychological Association (APA) explained that adults (42%) reported that they were not doing enough to manage their stress and some reported (20%) that they were not doing anything to manage their stress.[2] In the 2022 survey, 27% of Americans reported that they were so stressed that they could not function.[3] Stress was reported to impact the health of 76% of the adults. The symptoms experienced were "headache (38%), fatigue (35%), feeling nervous or anxious (34%), feeling depressed or sad (33%), and 72% experience feelings of being overwhelmed (33%), changes in sleep habits (32%), and constant worry (30%)."[4]

A review of yoga philosophy is the backdrop for the healing practices provided in this section. Instructions for teaching four breathing practices (pranayama), 22 yoga postures (asana), five hand gestures (mantras), and meditation (dhyana) are included in this section. Anatomy and physiology are not addressed in this book but there is a list of resources at the end of the book that have influenced the practices of the authors; not a fully inclusive list of all the works available but it provides a place to start. A few of the practitioner authors below are included in the list of resources and, among others, they provide a wealth of information and guidance.

- Anatomy: Susi Hately Aldous, David Coulter, Leslie Kaminoff and Amy Matthews, Ray Long, MD, Auturo Peal, and Mark Stephens, MD

- Meditation: Tara Bach, PhD, Ram Dass, Shelly Harrell, PhD, Dharma Khalsa, MD, Jack Kornfield

- Philosophy: Deborah Adele, Nischala Joy Devi, Eknath Easwaran, Georg Feuerstein, PhD, Maetreyii Ma Nolan, PhD, Roopa Pai, Shyam Ranganathan, PhD, Mark Whitwell

- Postures: Diane Bondy, Marsha Danzig, Mindy Eisenberg, Loren Fishman, MD, Judith Lasater, Timothy McCall, MD, David Frawley, Gail Parker, PhD, Mark Stephens, MD, Amy Weintraub

- Self-care: Queen Afual, Indu Arora, Shelly Harrell, PhD, Dharma Khalsa, MD, Vasant Lad, MASc, Gail Parker, PhD

- Yoga nidra: Indu Arora, Kamini Desai, PhD, Uma Dinsmore-Tuli, PhD, Richard Miller, PhD, Swami Satyananda Saraswati, Tracee Stanley

Another helpful resource is the Yoga Toolbox created by Joseph LePage and Lilian Aboim.[5] It includes an introduction to yoga philosophy, aspects of the individual (koshas) and physiological systems (muscular, skeletal, respiratory, circulatory, digestive, urinary, lymphatic, and excretory), yoga postures (asana), and much more.

CHAPTER 11

Yoga as a Healing Practice

Beginning yoga teachers should have a basic understanding of yoga philosophy. The philosophy provides a framework for understanding the yogic lifestyle, the physical practice of yoga, and informs the way that yoga is practiced and taught. By including these principles in how yoga is taught, the teacher can help students deepen their understanding and experience of yoga and also promote health, well-being, and spiritual growth.

Yoga is a spiritual and philosophical system that is both a way of life and a physical practice. Its aims are to promote physical, mental, and spiritual health and well-being. The Vedas (1700–1100 BCE) are thought to be the original source of yoga. They are composed of poems that explore consciousness and yoking the mind and the Divine. After the Vedic period, the Upanishads, written in the first millennium BCE, presented philosophical dialogue known as the end of the Vedas. The Bhagavad Gita addresses three paths to yoga:[1]

1. karma yoga: yoga of service

2. jnana yoga: yoga of knowledge

3. bhakti yoga: yoga of devotion.

Each of these paths extends far beyond the yoga mat and they can also impact how you teach yoga. Mark Stephens, MD, stated that a commitment to teaching yoga can be karmic service.[2] Jnana yoga is a practice of self-examination that leads to clarity that can benefit teacher and students. If bhakti yoga is the chosen path, connection with spiritual guides can be imparted to students.

The Yoga Sutras of Patanjali were composed around 200 CE and elaborate on the Bhagavad Gita. The Sutras introduce the path of raja yoga, the yoga of the mind, and describe a practice centered on steadying the mind. Interestingly, the beginning states of yoga are ethical and spiritual observations, not physical postures (asana). Foundationally, yoga is based on several key principles: ashtanga yoga, the *gunas*, law of karma, concept of dharma, the five elements, and the concept of self-realization.

The eight limbs As we discussed in Parts I and III, the eight limbs of yoga, known as ashtanga yoga, are a system of practices designed to promote spiritual growth and self-realization. The limbs are comprised of moral codes (yama), personal observances (niyama), postures (asana), breath control (pranayama), drawing the senses inward through releasing external distractions (pratyahara), concentration (dharana), meditation (dhyana), and oneness with the Divine (samadhi).

The *gunas* This philosophy of yoga recognizes three fundamental qualities of nature that are called *gunas*. The three qualities are *sattva* (purity, lightness, and harmony), *rajas* (activity, restlessness, and passion), and *tamas* (inertia, darkness, and ignorance). The *gunas* influence our physical, mental, and emotional states. As we navigate these states and can cultivate *sattva*, a state of balance and harmony can be achieved.

The law of karma This principle is an idea that every action that we take has a consequence, and that the consequences shape our lives and destinies. In yoga philosophy, karma is not only about cause and effect, it is also about the intention behind our actions, and how they impact ourselves and others.

The concept of dharma The principle of dharma is the idea of living in accordance with one's true nature or purpose, and fulfilling one's duties and responsibilities in life. According to yoga philosophy, living a life of dharma requires self-awareness, self-discipline, and a commitment to doing what is right. In *Radical Dharma: Talking Race, Love, and Liberation*, Sensei Angel Kyodo Williams, a Black activist and ordained Zen priest, Lama Owens, and Jasmine Syedullah, PhD, explore "the ever-present possibility of personal liberation and the resulting resilience, depth of capacity, peace of mind, strength of heart, and wise action."[3]

The five elements The philosophy of yoga and ayurveda recognizes five fundamental elements that make up the universe and all living beings.

These elements are earth, water, fire, air, and ether. Each element has its own qualities and characteristics and, by understanding these elements, we can better understand ourselves and our place in the world.

The concept of self-realization or recognition of true nature as a spiritual being is the ultimate goal of yoga philosophy. Self-realization is achieved through a process of self-inquiry and self-awareness, and by cultivating qualities such as compassion, wisdom, and detachment from that which deters this cultivation.

Modern interpretations of yoga were discussed in Part III. Mark Whitwell explains in his book, *Yoga of Heart: The Healing Power of Intimate Connection*, that the early teachers such as Yogananda and Shivananda that brought yoga to the West were more religious men than yogis.[4] They taught yoga techniques as a method of attaining spiritual goals. The focus on the principles of yoga varied for other modern teachers. As an example, B.K.S. Iyengar's form of yoga grew from his interest in "gymnastic anatomy" and for K. Phattabhi Jois his interest in "asana sequences." T.K.V. Desikachar "minimized *asana* and emphasized yoga as therapy, giving authority to Vedic scripture, Patanjali, and the teacher as a solution."[5]

Beginning yoga teachers should have a basic understanding of yoga philosophy. The philosophy provides a framework for understanding the yogic lifestyle, the physical practice of yoga, and informs the way that yoga is practiced and taught. By including these principles in how yoga is taught, the teacher can help students deepen their understanding and experience of yoga and also promote health, well-being, and spiritual growth.

In the West yoga classes can often be approached as a form of exercise, to get a good sweat, to outperform a friend, or even as a competition with oneself. However, a mindful yoga teacher inspires, creates safe and nurturing practices, encourages students to explore, and cultivates and broadens experiences and all aspects of the practice.

Prior to leading a class, take time to experience your own self-care practice. Then approach the class from a grounded space having prepared yourself to teach. Create your own self-care practice (*abhyasa*) or personal ritual (*dinacharya*) that you can practice before and after teaching yoga classes. The rituals can consist of activities that help you improve or maintain your own physical and mental health. According to the National Institute of Mental Health (NIMH), self-care helps to manage stress, decrease the risk of illness, and increases energy.[6] The NIMH recommendations include: (1) getting regular exercise; (2) eating healthy, regular meals and staying hydrated; (3) prioritizing sleep; (4) practicing gratitude; (5) focusing on positivity; (6) being connected with community; and (7) setting priorities and goals. Interestingly, these recommendations are very similar to ayurvedic and yoga lifestyle practices.

CHAPTER 12

How to Teach
Breathing Practices

*There are healing breath practices that everyone can do that can
activate the body's natural healing processes and connect one to self.*

Breathing is an important part of a yoga practice and, as the eight limbs
of yoga indicate, breathing practices/breath control (pranayama) are
practices in themselves and can be a precursor to and part of other
practices such as postures (asana) and meditation. Conscious breathing
opens one's mind, body, and spirit but that consciousness can slip away
if the awareness of the breath is not maintained.[1]

In the book, *The Healing Power of the Breath*, Richard Brown, MD,
and Patricia Gerbarg, MD, ask the question, "What do Mahatma Gandhi,
the martial artist Bruce Lee, Buddhist meditators, Christian monks,
Hawaiian *kahuna*, and...Special Forces have in common?"[2] Each uses
breathing to improve the quality of their well-being, physically, mentally,
and spiritually. There are healing breath practices that everyone can do
that can activate the body's natural healing processes and connect one to
self. While the practices can be healing, they take time. Timothy McCall,
MD, states in the book *Yoga as Medicine: The Yogic Prescription for Health
and Healing* that we learn yoga by doing.[3] "Yoga is not a panacea, but it
is a powerful medicine." It takes practice. It is slow medicine.

The breath is important physiologically. It is regulated involuntarily
through the central nervous system.[4] We breathe in and out automatically 24 hours a day and most of us do not have to think about it. There
are two types of breathing—costal (rib breathing) and diaphragmatic
(belly breathing).[5] In costal breathing, the ribs expand on the inhalation
(*purchaka*) and contract on the exhalation (*rechaka*). With diaphragmatic

breathing, the abdomen expands on the inhalation (*purchaka*) and contracts on the exhalation (*rechaka*). Seventy-five percent of breathing activities are due to diaphragmatic breathing.

A complete breath consists of inhalation, the space/suspension between the inhalation and the exhalation, exhalation, and the space/suspension between the inhalation and the exhalation.

Inhalation—*Purchaka*

Exhalation—*Rechaka*

Suspension—*Kumbhaka*

Suspension after the inhalation—*Antara kumbhaka*

Suspension after the exhalation—*Bahya kumbhaka*

Breathing also affects the sympathetic and parasympathetic nervous systems of the autonomic nervous system. Exhalations activate the parasympathetic nervous system and other systems such as respiratory, digestive, excretory, and circulatory systems. In addition to breath practices during yoga classes, encourage students to have their own regular breath practices. Focus on the natural breath, whether practicing breathing (pranayama) with or without postures (asana).

Diaphragmatic/full/three part breathing (*Dirga*)
dirga (slow, deep, long, complete)
Teach at the beginning of the practice.

Purpose: Increase breath awareness, expand lung capacity, and improve oxygen intake.

Cautions: None

Duration: 3–5 minutes

Rounds: 5–10 rounds

Cues to guide students: In an easy seated posture (*sukhasana*) or seated comfortably in a chair, with hands resting on the thighs or knees, supine (reclining) with legs extended or knees flexed, or standing in mountain (*tadasana*) observe the breathing without changing the breath. Notice the flow of breath in and out and the natural pauses between each breath. With eyes closed or with a soft gaze downward, inhale, noticing the abdomen expanding out, the ribcage expanding, and the upper chest expanding out. Exhale starting with the upper chest contracting inward, then the ribcage, and then the abdomen. Continue for several breaths with a slow, calm pattern. Return to natural breathing. Observe the changes in breathing quality or state of mind.

Highlight: Ease and steadiness. Stay relaxed and comfortable.

Modifications: When exhaling rest hands on the abdomen, ribcage, or upper chest to feel the breath in that area.

Alternate nostril breathing (*Nadi shodhana*)
nadi (channel) + *shodana* (cleaning, purifying)
+ pranayama (rhythmic yogic breathing)
Teach at the beginning of the practice.

Purpose: Balance and strengthen. Improve lung function and lower heart rate and blood pressure, and activate parasympathetic response. Increase concentration and prepare the body and mind for retention (*kumbhaka*). Activate and balance yin (*chandra*) and yang (*surya*) energies.

Cautions: Avoid retention for pregnancy, uncontrolled high blood pressure, heart disease, pressure inside the head, eye condition, and diabetes.

Duration: 3–5 minutes

Rounds: 5–10 rounds

Cues to guide students: In an easy seated posture (*sukhasana*) or seated comfortably in a chair, with hands resting on the thighs or knees, or standing in mountain (*tadasana*) observe the breathing without changing the breath. Notice the flow of breath in and out and the pauses between each breath. Begin diaphragmatic (*dirgha*) breathing with eyes closed or with a soft gaze downward for several breaths. Using the right hand, place the right thumb over the right nostril and the last two fingers over the left nostril. Close the left nostril with the last two fingers. Using even pressure on the left nostril, exhale completely through the right nostril. Close the right nostril with the right thumb and inhale slowly though the left nostril. Press the left nostril closed with the last two fingers and exhale with the right nostril, then inhale with the right nostril. Breathing through both nostrils is one full breath or one round. Close the left nostril with the last two fingers and exhale through the right nostril and continue another round. Breathe a comfortable ratio of 1:1 (inhalation [*purchaka*]:exhalation [*rechaka*]) or 1:1:1 (inhalation [*purchaka*]:retention [*antara kumbhaka*]:exhalation [*rechaka*]). Return to natural breathing. Observe the changes in breathing, quality, or state of mind.

Highlight: Ease and steadiness. Stay relaxed and comfortable.

Modifications: If there is stiffness, inflammation, or locking (e.g., trigger finger) in the fingers, the index and middle fingers can rest between the eyebrows.

Ratio breathing (*Sama-vritti* [equal fluctuation, sama-vee-ree-tee] and *Vi-sama-vritti* [unequal fluctuation, vee-sama vee-ree-tee])

sama (balanced, equal), *vi-sama* (imbalance, unequal) + *vritti* (modification) + pranayama (rhythmic yogic breathing)

Teach with natural breathing and *ujjayi*.

Purpose: Calm the mind. Inhalation (*purchaka*):retention (*antara kumbhaka*):exhalation (*rechaka*). Beginner—1:1:1 ratio; Intermediate—1:2:1; Advanced—1:4:1, 1:4:2.

Cautions: Avoid retention for pregnancy, uncontrolled high blood pressure, heart disease, pressure inside the head, eye condition and, diabetes, otherwise practice a 1:1 ratio.

Duration: 3–5 minutes

Rounds: 3–4 rounds, build up to 6–10 rounds

Cues to guide students: In an easy seated posture (*sukhasana*) or seated comfortably in a chair, with hands resting on the thighs or knees, or standing in mountain (*tadasana*) observe the breathing without changing the breath. Notice the flow of breath in and out and the pauses between each breath. Begin diaphragmatic (*dirgha*) breathing with eyes closed or with a soft gaze downward for several breaths. Inhale for the count of three while sensing the belly expand. Suspend the breath after the inhalation for a count of three and maintain the abdominal expansion. Exhale for a count of three observing the abdomen moving toward the spine and suspend the breath for a count of three. Repeat for the preferred number of rounds. Return to natural breathing. Observe the changes in breathing, quality, or state of mind.

Highlight: Ease and steadiness. Stay relaxed and comfortable.

Modifications: None

Victorious breath (*Ujjayi*)
ujjayi (to be victorious) + pranayama (rhythmic yogic breathing)
Teach at the beginning of class.

Purpose: Maintain focus and encourage energetic flow. Warms the breath by breathing through the nose only, warms the lungs, blood, and body. Sound and sensation help maintain awareness of the flow of the breath, rhythmic sound helps calm the nervous system. Inhalation (*purchaka*):retention (*antara kumbhaka*):exhalation (*rechaka*). Beginner—1:1:1 ratio; Intermediate—1:2:1; Advanced—1:4:1, 1:4:2.

Cautions: Avoid retention for pregnancy, uncontrolled high blood pressure, heart disease, pressure inside the head, eye condition and diabetes, otherwise practice a 1:1 ratio.

Duration: 3–5 minutes and during practice when appropriate

Rounds: 3–4 rounds, build up to 6–10 rounds

Cues to guide students: In an easy seated posture (*sukhasana*) or seated comfortably in a chair, with hands resting on the thighs or knees, or standing in mountain (*tadasana*). Observe the breathing without changing the breath. Notice the flow of breath in and out and the pauses between each breath. Begin diaphragmatic (*dirgha*) breathing with eyes closed or with a soft gaze downward for several breaths. Breathe through the nose, slightly closing off the back of the throat at the epiglottis. Experience the same sound and sensation on the inhalation (*purchaka*) and the exhalation (*rechaka*). After several rounds return to natural breathing. Observe the changes in breathing, quality, or state of mind.

Highlight: Ease and steadiness. Stay relaxed and comfortable. Be gentle with the breath and do not overly restrict the breath.

Modifications: None

CHAPTER 13

How to Teach Yoga Postures (Asanas)

...be fully present for those "in the room" whether in person or virtual.

The yoga class that you teach is not your yoga practice! It is a time to be fully present for those "in the room" whether in person or virtual, indoors or outdoors, on a mat or in a chair. Be observant throughout the class. Take a few moments to greet participants, check in with them, and offer the opportunity, in a non-attributable way, to share with the teacher if they have medical conditions or injuries that day that they want to honor. And then be aware of this input throughout the class and provide guidance with this in mind.

Farhi and Stuart, in their book *Pathways to a Centered Body*, suggest that practitioners do "a little body weather reading at the beginning of each practice session."[1] This weather reading helps practitioners become aware of changes (interoception) when they compare what they experience during and after classes to their "weather condition" at the beginning of the practice. The process is useful for practitioners to be able to discern what practices are beneficial in mitigating their current state and any uneasiness or suffering that they might be experiencing.

The growing interest in holistic health and well-being addresses individuals from a perspective of mind, body, and spirit. The yoga and whole person perspectives sometimes referred to as biopsychosocial consider alignment of the yogic perspective of sheaths/levels (kosha)— the physical body (*sthula*), the subtle body (*sukshma*), and the causal body (*karana*).

The koshas can be further described starting from the periphery moving inward, the physical level (anamaya kosha), inward to the subtle body—energy level (pranamaya kosha), emotions (manomaya kosha), and intellect (vijnanamaya kosha), and the spirit/bliss/causal body (anandamaya kosha). Present inquiries related to these levels/sheaths (kosha) and encourage participants to conduct personal inquiry and reflection such as:

1. What are they experiencing in the physical body? (physical—anamaya kosha)

2. What is the energy level that they are experiencing? What is the breath like? (breath/energy—pranamaya kosha)

3. What emotions are present and how do those emotions show up for them? (mind—manomaya kosha)

4. How are their spirits? Reflect on what gives them meaning. (intellect—vijnanamaya kosha; spiritual—anandamaya kosha)

When teaching, start with the least ambitious postures so that students can warm up, be successful in safe positions, and prepare for more challenging postures (asana) if that is their interest. Notice if a student appears to be confused or struggling. Offer modifications and variations to everyone, so that students can choose how they want to express the posture (asana) without feeling called out as not being able to meet someone else's expectations of what the posture (asana) should look like. By offering these options to everyone, students can learn to be attuned to what is appropriate for themselves.

Yoga postures (asana) are preparation for the practices of pranayama, dharana, dhyana, and samadhi. In her book *Yoga* Indu Arora explains that there are four important considerations of asana: action, purpose, position, and movement.[2] Reflect on action, purpose, position, and movement for the practice overall and for each posture (asana). Consider including six movements of the body (contraction, stretch, twist, forward bend, back bend, and lateral stretch) in each practice or class. These five movements are also important for the health of the spine.[3]

Contraction stimulates the release of metabolic waste. Stretching lengthens muscles, increases the cellular surface so that they can absorb oxygen, and increases flexibility. Twisting stimulates cellular metabolism, and forward bending calms the nervous system by activating the parasympathetic nervous system. Back bending increases circulation and flexibility, and lateral stretching lengthens muscles and creates spaces for the internal organs.[4] Farhi and Stuart created a six-step protocol to "build cognitive and experiential understanding" of the psoas muscles, deep core muscles that, along with the gluteus maximus and piriformis, connect the torso and lower body.[5] Conceptually, this protocol can also be applied to the practice overall: (1) know what body part is involved; (2) warm up and hydrate the body; (3) release and lengthen muscles and fascia (include diaphragmatic breathing); (4) balance sides (applies to sides of the body as well as agonist and antagonist muscles); (5) strengthen; (6) move from a core integration maintaining "good posture and movement alignment."

Have a good flow in mind when planning what to teach in a class. Consider how to purposefully guide students through an experience for their own journeys. The foundation for creating a class could begin with a seated meditation and breathing practice, initial warm up, standing postures, abdominals (option), balance postures, back bending postures, twisting postures, inversions, and ending in rest.

The following postures (asana) provide examples of the aforementioned considerations and movements. Read through the information provided for each posture (asana) and get a sense of the depth of each posture (asana). These postures (asana) were selected because they could be helpful for many of the conditions listed in Part II by incorporating the appropriate modification and/or variation for the individual practicing the posture (asana). Some postures (asana) are appropriate for restorative practices and some variations can be appropriate for practitioners interested in a more vigorous practice.

Back bend postures (asana)

Bridge—*Setu bandhasana*
Cobra—*Bhujangasana*
Locust—*Salabhasana*

Balancing postures (asana)/Stabilization

Bridge—*Setu bandhasana*
Extended side angle—*Utthita parsvakonasana*
Half moon/Side extension—*Ardha chandrasana*
Mountain/Equal standing—*Tadasana*

Plank/Four-limbed—*Chaturanga dandasana*
Tree—*Vrksasana*
Triangle—*Utthita trikonasana*
Warrior 1—*Virabhadrasana 1*

Inversion postures (asana)

Bridge—*Setu bandhasana*
Downward-facing dog—*Adho mukha svanasana*
Legs up the wall—*Viparita karani*

Prone postures (asana)

Cat–Cow/Table—*Marjariasana/Sandharasan/Bharmanasana*
Child's—*Balasana*
Cobra—*Bhujangasana*
Locust—*Salabhasana*
Plank/Four-limbed—*Chaturanga dandasana*

Restorative postures (asana)

Bridge—*Setu bandhasana*
Child's—*Balasana*
Corpse—*Savasana*
Legs up the wall—*Viparita karani*

Seated postures (asana)

Easy seated—*Sukhasana*
Seated spinal twist/Half Lord of the Fishes posture—*Ardha matsy-endrasana*
Staff—*Dandasana*

Standing postures (asana)

Chair—*Utkatasana*
Extended side angle—*Utthita parsvakonasana*
Half moon/Side extension—*Ardha chandrasana*
Mountain/Equal standing—*Tadasana*
Tree—*Vrksasana*
Triangle—*Utthita trikonasana*
Warrior 1—*Virabhadrasana 1*
Warrior 2—*Virabhadrasana 2*

Supine postures (asana)

Bridge—*Setu bandhasana*
Corpse—*Savasana*
Knee to chest/Wind release—*Apanasana*
Legs up the wall—*Viparita karani*

POSTURES (ASANA)

Bridge—*Setu bandhasana (SET-too bahn-DAHS-anna)*
setu (dam, bridge) + *bandha* (lock) + asana (posture)

Category: Supine, back bend

Benefits: Strengthens the back. Lengthens/opens the front body. Extends the spine.

Cautions: Uncontrolled high blood pressure, glaucoma, hiatal, umbilical, and inguinal hernias, stroke history, migraine. Neck, shoulder, back, and knee issues.

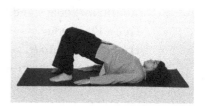

FIGURE 13.1 BRIDGE POSE, SUPINE VARIATION, SIDE VIEW.

Cues to guide students: Lie on the back, bend the knees with feet on the floor and ankles aligned with the knees. Legs are hip-width apart. Place arms alongside the body with shoulders away from the ears and palms on the floor. Keep the spine long and engage the middle and lower trapezius to draw the shoulders toward

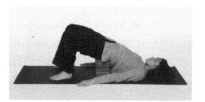

FIGURE 13.2 BRIDGE POSE, SUPINE VARIATION WITH YOGA BLOCKS, SIDE VIEW.

the hips. Feet press against the floor to lift the hips. Brace the torso, exhale and lift the hips and spine from the floor. Exhale to return to the floor and repeat several times then lift and hold for several breaths.

Highlight: Internal rotation of thigh bone (femur). Press down through feet and shoulders. Broaden across chest.

Modifications:

▸ Place a strap around the ankles, holding one end in each hand. Lift the hips from the floor.

▸ Place a block between the thighs, pressing the thighs together to hold the block and lift the hips from the floor.

Variations:

▸ Practice pelvic tilts prior for expressing bridge (*setu bandhasana*). Inhale pressing the sacrum into the floor and arch the back. Exhale pressing the tailbone (sacrum) against the floor.

▶ Lift the hips, placing in the hands under the sacrum or buttocks with fingers extended to support the hips.

▶ Lift the hips, extend one leg toward the ceiling, pressing the sole of the foot or ball of the foot toward the ceiling. The hands can be clasped beneath the body with arms extended or can support the hips. Release and switch legs.

▶ Lift the hips, placing the hands under the sacrum for support, both legs are extended with feet on the floor.

Restorative: Place a block, bolster, or rolled blanket under the sacrum. Release the body to the block, bolster, or rolled blanket and relax.

Cat–Cow—*Marjariasana* (MAR-ja-ri-AHS-anna)/ *Sandharasana* (san-DHAR-as-anna)/ Table—*Bharmanasana* (BHAR-maa-NAS-anna)
marjari (cat) + asana (posture)/*sandhara* (table) + asana (posture)/*bharman* (table top) + asana (posture)

Category: Stabilization

Benefits: Cultivates spinal flexibility and stability. Strengthens wrists, elbows, hips, and knees. Massages organs. Encourages balance and grounding. With table pose (*bharmanasana*) extension and balancing, stretches hips, core, thighs, knees, and spine.

Cautions: Wrist and hand issues, use a wedge or rolled blanket. Hyper-flexible elbows, slightly flex elbows.

Cues to guide students: Start on hands and knees with wrists aligned with shoulders and knees aligned with hips. Press the palms into the floor with fingers spread wide. Release shoulders away from the ears. Press the hands onto the floor and slightly rotate the crease of the elbows in the same direction as the fingers. Engage the core for a neutral lumbar curve. Lengthen the spine. Hold this table pose (*bharmanasana*) for a few breaths. Exhale rounding the back by pressing the tailbone down, chin toward the chest. Inhale lifting the tailbone, lower the chest toward the floor and lift the head. Continue moving with the breath.

Highlight: Press down through feet and shoulders.

Modifications:

▸ Place a folded blanket under the knees.

▸ Place a foam wedge or rolled blanket on the mat to support the wrists and hands.

▸ Place forearms on blocks to ease the pressure on the wrists and hands.

▸ Place a strap around the thighs and press out into the strap.

▸ Place a block between the thighs and press into the block.

Variations:

▸ Place the forearms on the floor with elbows aligned with the shoulders.

▸ Add lateral movement by moving the shoulder and hip on the same side toward each other with the breath.

▸ Vary the placement of the hands.

Chair—*Utkatasana* (OOT-kah-TAHS-anna)
utkata (awkward) + asana (posture)

Category: Standing, stabilization

Benefits: Strengthens and stabilizes the joints. Builds digestive fire.

Cautions: Ankle, knee, hip, or back issues. Practice modifications during pregnancy.

Cues to guide students: Standing in mountain, ground all four corners of the feet. Raise the arms in front to shoulder height with palms turned toward each other. Activate the core, lift the kneecaps, maintain a neutral spine, and bend the knees lowering the hips as if sitting in a chair. Relax the

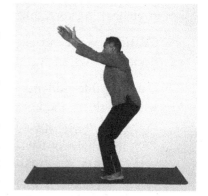

FIGURE 13.3 CHAIR POSE, STANDING VARIATION, SIDE VIEW.

shoulders. The torso hinges forward slightly. Keep the thighs active by visualizing pressing out into an imaginary strap around the thighs.

Highlight: Keep chest open. Lengthen the spine. Activate the legs.

Modifications:

▸ Stand with the back against the wall with knees and ankles aligned.

▸ Place a block between the thighs, with back against wall or standing.

▸ Lie on back with feet pressed against the wall with knees flexed at 90 degrees and ankles aligned with knees, with or without a block between thighs.

Variations:

▸ Standing with arms overhead aligned with ears.

▸ Standing with fingers interlaced and palms turned outward, arms extended in front or overhead.

▸ With hands in prayer position (*anjali mudra*) in front of the heart, rotate outside of the elbow to the outside of the opposite knee.

▸ Chair with a twist pose—with hand in prayer position (*anjali mudra*) in front of the heart, place an elbow to the outside of the opposite thigh. Return to chair (*utkatasana*) and repeat on the other side.

Vinyasa:

▸ Inhale in mountain pose, exhale to chair pose. Inhale return to mountain pose.

▸ Inhale in chair, exhale flexing at

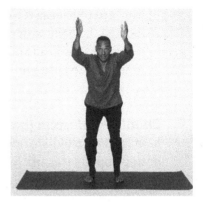

FIGURE 13.4 CHAIR POSE, STANDING VARIATION, FRONT VIEW.

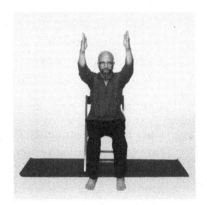

FIGURE 13.5 CHAIR POSE, SEATED VARIATION, FRONT VIEW.

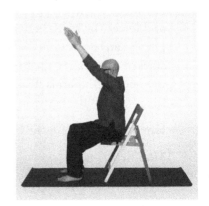

FIGURE 13.6 CHAIR POSE, SEATED VARIATION, SIDE VIEW.

the hip so that the torso is parallel to the floor, extend the arms behind the body with palms facing the ceiling, each other, or the floor. The head and spine are in natural extension. Inhale returning to chair with arms in a preferred position.

Child's—*Balasana* (bah-LAHS-anna)
bala (young, childish, not fully grown or developed) + asana (posture)

Category: Prone

Benefits: Hip and knee flexion. Gentle spinal traction. Massages the abdominal organs, supporting digestion and elimination. Facilitates circulation to the head, senses, and brain. Calms the nervous system. Cultivates safety and calmness.

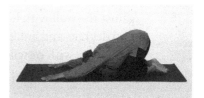

FIGURE 13.7 CHILD'S POSE, PRONE VARIATION, SIDE VIEW.

Cautions: Low back, knees, pregnancy.

Cues to guide students: From table posture (*sandharasana/bharmanasana*) place the tops of the feet on the floor, beginning with knees hip-width apart. Lower the hips to the heels and abdomen to the thighs with forearms on the floor. For more comfort, open the knees out and lower the torso between the knees.

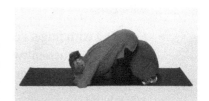

FIGURE 13.8 CHILD'S POSE, PRONE VARIATION WITH BOLSTER, SIDE VIEW.

Hands can be positioned with palms facing the ceiling or on the floor, or stacked fists resting the forehead on the stacked hands, arms alongside the body with hands near the feet, palms up or palms down. Release the weight of the body.

Highlight: Stay with the breath, relaxation within.

Modifications:

▶ Place a rolled towel or blanket behind the knees.

▶ Place a rolled towel or blanket between the floor and tops of the ankles.

▶ Open knees apart with big toes touching.

Variations:

▸ Extended child's pose: extend arms past ears with palms on the floor, press back through tailbone.

▸ Extended child's pose with arm variations.

▸ Lift hips high enough to find comfort.

▸ Arms extended in front, walk the hands to the left and hold for a few breaths. Walk hands back to center and repeat on the other side.

Vinyasa:

▸ Exhale to child's pose (*balasana*) and inhale returning to table (*sandharasana/bharmanasana*). Repeat for several breaths and return to table (*sandharasana/bharmanasana*) or rest in child's pose (*balasana*).

Restorative: Place a blanket as desired beneath the knees, bolster between the back of the legs, rolled blanket between tops of the feet and the mat, resting the forehead on a pillow, block, or stacked hands. Another option is to rest the hands alongside the body.

Cobra—*Bhujangasana* (boo-jang-GAHS-anna)
bhujanga (serpent)/*bhuja* (arm, shoulder) +
anga (limb) + asana (posture)

Category: Prone, back bend

Benefits: Strengthens and lengthens the back. Stretches the front of the torso. Supports digestion and elimination.

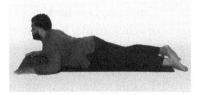

FIGURE 13.9 COBRA POSE, PRONE VARIATION, SIDE VIEW.

Cautions: Low back, hyperextended neck, inguinal hernia, pregnancy, back issues, uncontrolled high blood pressure, heart disease, or a history of stroke.

Cues to guide students: Lying prone on the abdomen with legs extended and feet hip-width apart, extend arms overhead, palms on the floor, and forehead resting on the floor. Engage the core and lengthen the spine.

Flex the elbows and place hands on the floor aligned with the shoulders, fingers apart. The upper arms hug the sides of the ribcage. Hands pressing forward, inhaling, ground the pelvis, legs, and feet. Lengthen the spine, lift the chest and head using back strength. Release back to the floor on the exhalation. Repeat with the breath several times and either hold for a few breaths or release and rest.

Modifications:

▸ Place a bolster or rolled blanket underneath the body lengthwise between the pubic bone and the throat notch.

Variations:

▸ For upward-facing dog (*urdhva mukha svanasa*) press the tops of the feet to lift the legs and pelvis from the floor. The gaze (drishti) is forward.

Corpse—*Savasana* (shah-VAHS-anna)
savo/shava (corpse) + asana (posture)

Category: Supine, final relaxation

Benefits: Balances all body systems, especially the nervous, endocrine, and digestive. Beneficial for stress, high blood pressure, and, for some people, anxiety. Cultivates deep relaxation.

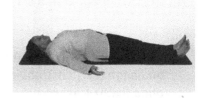

FIGURE 13.10 CORPSE POSE, SUPINE VARIATION, SIDE VIEW.

Cautions: Low back, depression, anxiety, or other mental health conditions should begin with movement prior to *savasana*. During pregnancy, an option is to lie on the side rather than supine.

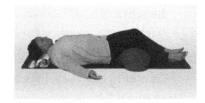

FIGURE 13.11 CORPSE POSE, SUPINE VARIATION WITH BOLSTER, SIDE VIEW.

Cues to guide students: Lie supine with bent knees and feet on the floor (constructive rest) or legs extended slightly out from hip-width apart. Arms are alongside the body with palms turned up and shoulders down away from ears. Tuck the chin slightly. Relax the body.

Highlight: Neck is long and relaxed. Neutral spine/low back.

Modifications:

▶ Place a bolster, rolled blanket, or blocks under the knees.

▶ Small roll under the neck and/or ankles.

▶ If side lying, blanket between the knees and the head to maintain spinal alignment.

Variations:

▶ For constructive rest lie on the back with knees bent, feet on the floor, and arms alongside the body.

Restorative: Sometimes called mountain brook. Use all of the modifications listed above. Gently cover the eyes with an eye pillow or some other lightweight material. Arms alongside the body. Support wrists if desired. Another option is to prop the student up with blocks and bolsters.

Downward-facing dog—*Adho mukha svanasana* (ah-doh moo-kah shah-VAHS-anna)
adho (downward) + *mukha* (face)
+ *shvana* (dog) + asana (posture)

Category: Inversion, stabilization

Benefits: Lengthens and aligns the spine. Strengthens legs and arms. Integrates body, mind, and spirit.

Cautions: Ankle, wrist, elbow, shoulder, neck or spinal issues, pregnancy.

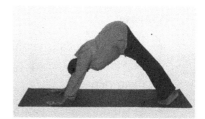

FIGURE 13.12 DOWNWARD-FACING DOG POSE, STANDING VARIATION, SIDE VIEW.

Cues to guide students: From table pose (*bharmanasana*), curl the toes under and on the exhalation lift the hips to extend the legs, maintaining knee flexion and pressing the sitting bones back and lengthening the spine through to the coccyx. Press wide-spread fingers into the floor and rotate the creases of the elbows forward slightly. Maintain head, neck, and spine alignment with the gaze

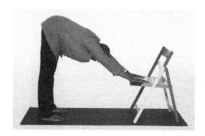

FIGURE 13.13 DOWNWARD-FACING DOG POSE, CHAIR VARIATION, SIDE VIEW.

(drishti) between the feet. Extend the legs unless the spine is rounding. In that case maintain a slight bend in the knees. Inhale returning to table (*bharmanasana*). This flow is helpful for warming up.

Highlight: Lift the thighs up. Head, neck, abdomen relaxed.

Modifications:

▶ Palms on the seat of a chair.

▶ Knees bent.

▶ "Walk" the feet, alternately lifting one heel at a time.

▶ Strap around the upper arms pressing the arms into the strap.

▶ Place a block between the thighs.

▶ Wedge under the wrists or the heels.

Variations:

▶ For three-legged dog, lift one leg upward, toes toward the floor, keeping the hips level.

▶ For dolphin pose (*ardha pincha mayurasana*), forearms are on the floor with the option to interlace fingers.

Vinyasa:

▶ From table pose (*bharmanasana*), exhale to downward-facing dog (*adho mukha svanasana*). Inhale to return to table pose (*bharmanasana*).

▶ From downward-facing dog (*adho mukha svanasana*), inhaling, lift one leg, exhaling, bring the knee toward the chest. Inhale extending the leg again. Repeat several cycles on one side and then switch sides or flow alternately from one leg to the other.

Easy seated—*Sukhasana* (suk-HAS-anna)
sukha (comfortable, gentle, agreeable) + asana (posture)

Category: Seated, hip opener

Benefits: Stretches knees and ankles, aligns the spine, sense of ease.

Cautions: Knees, groin, hips, lower spine, sciatica.

Cues to guide students: Seated on the floor, extend both legs. Flex both knees, tucking one foot under the opposite thigh. Ground through the sitting bones and extend the spine from the tailbone (sacrum) to the crown of the head.

Modifications:

▸ Sit on the edge of a folded blanket or bolster.

▸ Blocks or folded blanket beneath the outer thighs/knees.

▸ Back against a wall.

▸ Seated comfortably in a chair with soles of the feet on the floor or block(s).

Variations:

▸ Adjust the width of the legs based on comfort.

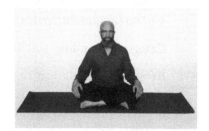

FIGURE 13.14 EASY SEATED POSE, SEATED VARIATION, FRONT VIEW.

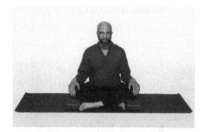

FIGURE 13.15 EASY SEATED POSE, SEATED VARIATION WITH BLOCKS, FRONT VIEW.

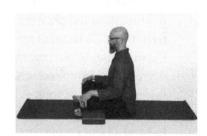

FIGURE 13.16 EASY SEATED POSE, SEATED VARIATION WITH BLOCKS, SIDE VIEW.

Extended side angle—*Utthita parsvakonasana* (oo-TEE-tah parsh-vah-ko-NAHS-anna)

utthita (extended) + *parsva/parshva* (side, flank) + *kona* (angle) *Parivritta* (rotated, twisted) + asana (posture)

Category: Standing, stabilization

Benefits: Circulation to the digestive, excretory, and reproductive systems. Stretches the intercostal muscles and expands breath capacity. Massages the lymph glands in the groin and armpits.

Cautions: Misaligned front knee, hyperextended back knee, shoulder impingement, low back. Neck if looking up. Shoulder impingement. Spinal disc or hip issues, pregnancy, uncontrolled hypertension, hernia, gastritis.

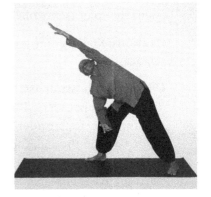

FIGURE 13.17 EXTENDED SIDE ANGLE POSE, STANDING VARIATION, FRONT VIEW.

Cues to guide students: From warrior 2 (*virabhadrasana 2*), keep the feet grounded. Reach out through the right fingertips, then flex the elbow and place the forearm on the front thigh. Or begin in a wide stance. Lift the front toes to turn the right foot out 90 degrees. The front heel is aligned with the instep of the back foot. Adjust the width of the stance for preference. Activate both legs and all four corners of the feet. Finding stability, hold for a few breaths with hips squared forward and hands on the waist. Flex front knee over the ankle. The thigh will be parallel to the floor. Flex the front elbow and place the forearm on

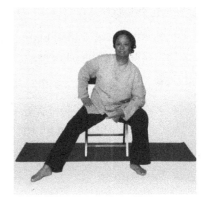

FIGURE 13.18 EXTENDED SIDE ANGLE POSE, SEATED VARIATION WITH CHAIR, FRONT VIEW.

the front thigh. Extend the back arm so that the upper arm is near the ear. Lengthen the torso to experience extension from the outside of the back ankle to the fingertips. Use the core muscles for stability rather than the arms. Draw the feet together isometrically. Hold for a few breaths then switch sides. Then, release to warrior 2 (*virabhadrasana 2*) or wide standing.

Highlight: Line from back foot through to extended arm fingertips. Ground back heel, weight on outside edges of both feet. Rotate hips, chest, shoulders, and top arm.

Modifications:

▸ Front arm extended with hand on a block in front of the instep.

▸ Front arm extended with hand on a block along the outside edge of the foot.

▸ Use a strap for the arm binding, an end of the strap in each hand without slack in the strap.

▸ Back facing the wall with the back heel at the wall.

▸ Facing the wall.

Variations:

▸ Back knee on the floor with body facing forward. The forward leg is flexed at the knee perpendicular to the back leg. Bear weight evenly on both legs.

▸ The variations below can be practiced standing or with one knee on the floor:

    – Gaze (drishti) down at the floor or up toward the ceiling.

    – Back arm with hand on the waist.

    – Back arm with forearm behind the back.

    – Bind the back arm behind the back. Front arm extends beneath the front thigh to grasp the hand of the back arm.

Vinyasa:

▸ Extend (straighten) and flex (bend) the front leg with the breath.

▸ Slowly gaze up and down with the breath.

▸ Flow from extended side angle (*utthita parsvakonasana*) to warrior 2 (*virabhadrasana 2*).

Half moon/Side extension—*Ardha chandrasana* (arh-dah chan-DRAHS-anna)
ardha (half) + *chandra* (moon) + asana (posture)

Category: Standing, lateral bend

Benefits: Promotes lateral spinal flexibility. Improves circulation to the liver, pancreas, spleen, and thymus gland. Strengthens legs and core.

Cautions: Neck, hyperextended knee, low back. Uncontrolled hypertension, lumbar disc and sacral issues.

Cues to guide students: Standing in mountain (*tadasana*) with feet hip-width apart and arms along the sides, activate the legs and core, and press the four corners of the feet against the floor. Inhale lifting the arms overhead, releasing the shoulders from the ears. Lengthen the spine and exhale arching to the side. Hold for a few breaths and repeat on the other side.

Highlight: External hip rotation, stability in the standing leg.

Modifications:

▸ Stand perpendicular to a wall and lean toward the wall for support.

▸ Back against a wall.

▸ Bottom hand on a block or chair.

Variations:

▸ Hands down alongside the body.

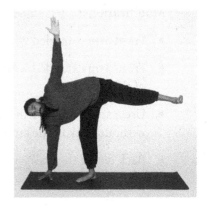

FIGURE 13.19 HALF MOON POSE, BALANCING VARIATION, FRONT VIEW.

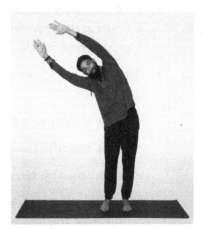

FIGURE 13.20 HALF MOON POSE, STANDING VARIATION, FRONT VIEW.

▸ Interlace fingers overhead.

▸ Lean to the side of a chair seat, block on the floor, or fingertips to the floor. Lift the opposite side leg parallel to the floor and extend through the heel.

▸ Seated (floor) half moon pose (*ardha chandrasana*) from easy seated pose (*sukhasana*), reach one arm overhead, bending laterally while pressing the opposite hand or forearm onto the floor.

▸ Seated (chair) half moon pose (*ardha chandrasana*) from easy seated pose (*sukhasana*), reach one arm overhead, bending laterally while extending the opposite hand toward the floor.

Vinyasa:

▸ Extend one arm overhead with the other hand pressing against the hip.

▸ Lengthen the low back and press the back against the wall.

▸ Half moon pose (*ardha chandrasana*) can also be practiced lying on the back, banana pose (*bananasana*).

▸ Exhale to one side and inhale back to center, moving with the breath.

▸ Extend arms overhead and interlace the fingers, rotating the palms upward.

▸ While bending laterally, draw the opposite hand up toward the armpit, moving with the breath from side to side.

Low lunge—*Anjaneyasana* (ahn-jon-un-YAHS-anna)
anjani (named after Hanuman) + asana (posture)

Category: Standing

Benefits: Stretches hip flexors, strengthens knees and core muscles. Improves focus and stability.

Cautions: Low back, neck, and knees.

Cues to guide students: From downward-facing dog (*adho mukha svanasana*), exhale stepping the right foot forward between the hands, aligning the right ankle with the right knee, thigh parallel to the floor. Lower the left knee to the floor placing the top of the left foot on the floor. Rest the hands on the floor on the sides of the right foot. Lengthen the spine and hold for a few breaths. Curling the left foot toes under, lift the back knee, and step the front foot back to downward-facing dog (*adho mukha svanasana*). Repeat low lunge (*anjaneyasana*) on the opposite side.

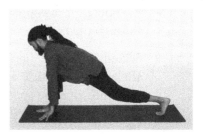

FIGURE 13.21 LOW LUNGE POSE, STANDING VARIATION, SIDE VIEW.

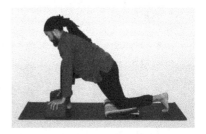

FIGURE 13.22 LOW LUNGE POSE, STANDING VARIATION WITH BLOCKS, SIDE VIEW.

Modifications:

▸ Pad or folded blanket under the back knee.

▸ Block on floor to inside or outside of front foot.

▸ Blocks on floor to the inside and outside of the front foot.

Variations:

▸ Vary hand positions from on the floor to the front thigh, in prayer position (*anjali mudra*), arms out, arms overhead in "V" or "Y" positions.

▸ From hand in prayer position (*anjali mudra*), inhaling, extend elbows out from center, exhaling, rotate upper torso to the direction of the front leg. Extend front arm in the direction of the front knee, and the other arm backward.

▶ From hand in prayer position (*anjali mudra*), inhaling, extend elbows out from center, exhaling, rotate upper torso to the direction of the front leg.

Knee-down twist—*Jathara parivartanasana* (ja-THA-ra pari-VAR-tan-NAS-anna)
jathara (abdomen, stomach) + *parivartana* (revolving) + asana (posture)
Vinyasa:

▶ Exhaling, sit back on the back heel, inhaling, return forward.

▶ Exhaling, sit back on the back heel and extend the front leg, inhaling, return forward.

▶ From an arm variation open/extend the arms on an inhalation, exhaling, bring arms back to center.

Knees-to-chest/Wind releasing—*Apanasana* (ah-pah-NAHS-anna)
apana (downward moving vital current of energy) + asana (posture)

Category: Supine, hip opener

Benefits: Massages the excretory, urinary, reproductive, and digestive systems. Stabilizes the pelvis. Releases low back tension. Calms the nervous system. Supports releasing what is not of service.

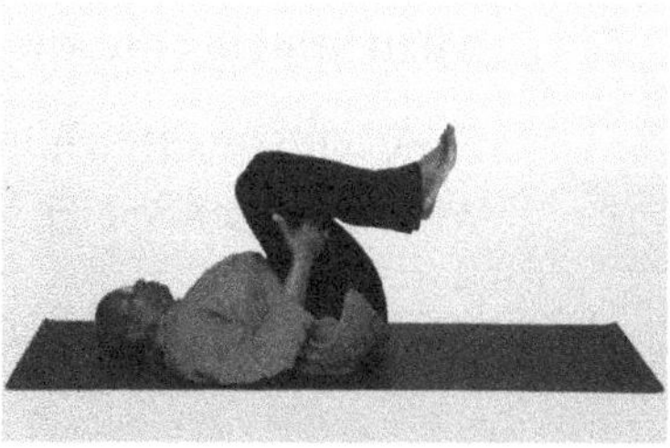

Cautions: Low back, knee, groin issues.

FIGURE 13.23 WIND RELEASING POSE, SUPINE VARIATION, SIDE VIEW.

Cues to guide students: Lying on the back, bend knees with feet on the floor hip-width apart. Arms are alongside the body with palms down. Engage core and slightly tuck the chin toward the chest. Keeping the tailbone (sacrum) grounded and the pelvis level, exhale bringing the knee in toward the chest. Place the palm, with interlaced fingers, on the shin, below the knee, or behind the thigh. The ankle is flexed. Release the shoulders from the ears. Hold for a few breaths, then switch legs.

Highlight: Be mindful of the low back. Avoid hyperextending the knee when extending the leg.

Modifications:

▸ One foot on the floor when bringing the opposite knee to the chest.

▸ A strap or scarf behind the thigh of the knee to the chest.

▸ Foot of extended leg on a wall.

▸ Block under the tailbone (sacrum) and gently press the ball of the extended foot into a wall.

▸ During pregnancy separate the knees to the side of the abdomen.

Variations:

▸ Lift the heel of the extended leg off the floor while moving the opposite knee to the chest.

▸ Lift forehead toward the knee to the chest. Ensure core muscles are engaged.

Vinyasa:

▸ Alternate knees to the chest moving with the breath. Exhaling when bringing the knees to the chest.

▸ Flow with breath while alternating bringing the knees to the chest with the extended leg lifted and forehead toward the knee.

Legs up the wall—*Viparita karani* (vip-pah-ree-tah kuh-RAHN-ee)

viparita (turned around, reversed, inverted) + *karani* (doing, making, action) + asana (posture)

Category: Inversion

Benefits: Tractions and aligns the spine. Increases circulation to the thyroid and thymus glands, brain, and face. Optimizes circulation to the lungs and digestive organs. Massages the kidneys and adrenal glands. Enhances venous return from the leg. Calms the nervous system.

Cautions: Hamstrings, low back.

Cues to guide students: In bridge pose (*setu bandhasana*) with the upper back on the floor, the knees are flexed with feet on the floor, ankles aligned with the knees, legs are hip-width apart, shoulders are released from the ears, and hips lifted, extend the arms underneath the torso. Lift the heels, coming onto the toes. Then lift the feet off the floor one at a time, bringing legs perpendicular to the floor. With the hands supporting the hips

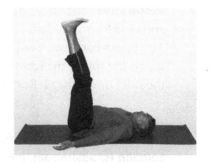

FIGURE 13.24 LEGS UP THE WALL POSE, SUPINE VARIATION, SIDE VIEW.

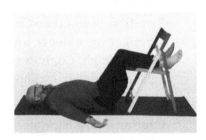

FIGURE 13.25 LEGS UP THE WALL POSE, SUPINE VARIATION WITH CHAIR, SIDE VIEW.

(pelvis), fingers pointed in the direction of the buttocks (gluteal muscles), the upper arms are on the floor with forearms perpendicular to the floor. The weight of the lower body is evenly distributed across the shoulders and upper arms. Press the hands toward the buttocks (glutes), engage the core muscles, and lengthen the legs toward the ceiling, drawing the thighs back into the hip socket. Hold for several breaths. Release one foot at a time back to the floor returning to bridge (*setu bandhasana*) and then back to the floor.

Highlight: Leg stability

Modifications:

▸ Strap around lower legs to hold legs together.

▸ Sandbag/book on the feet for stability.

▸ Block under the tailbone (sacrum).

▸ Arms can be alongside the body.

Restorative: Place a bolster/pillow horizontally at the wall. Sit at one end of the bolster, then lie back and swivel the legs up onto the wall. The upper back and head rest on the floor. A sandbag may be placed across the top of the feet to enhance grounding. The arms can rest by the sides or overhead. Rest here for 5–10 minutes.

Locust—*Salabhasana* (sha-la-BAHS-anna)
salabha (grasshopper, locust) + asana (posture)

Category: Prone, back bend

Benefits: Strengthens the back body. Massages the kidneys, and adrenal and thymus glands. Cultivates the balance of lightness and stability. Supports digestion and elimination.

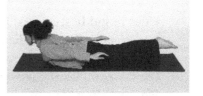

FIGURE 13.26 LOCUST POSE, PRONE VARIATION, SIDE VIEW.

Cautions: Low back, neck, shoulders if extending arms near ears, pregnancy, uncontrolled high blood pressure.

Cues to guide students: Lying prone on the abdomen, legs extended, and feet hip-width apart, rest the chin or forehead on the floor. The arms are alongside the body. Engage the core, press the pelvis into the floor or hands and draw the shoulders

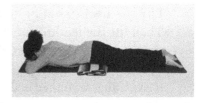

FIGURE 13.27 LOCUST POSE, PRONE VARIATION WITH BLANKET, SIDE VIEW.

away from the ears. Find half locust (*ardha salbhasana*) to warm up/ prepare for the full locust (*salbhasana*) posture, hug the upper arms to the ribs, flex the knee, inhale, and lift a leg to a comfortable height with the foot flexed using the strength of the buttock (gluteal muscles) and hamstring. Exhale and release back to the floor and repeat 3–4 times, then switch legs and repeat the movement with the opposite leg. For full locust (*salbhasana*) posture, re-engage the core, lift both legs from the floor, toes point away from the hips. Soften any tension in the neck, face, and jaw. Hold for several breaths, then release.

Modifications:

▶ Place a folded blanket or bolster under the thighs or pelvis.

Variations:

▶ For half locust posture (*ardha salbhasana*), align the spine, press the pelvis into the floor, engage the core muscles, flex both knees with the feet flexed, hands alongside the body, palms down, lift one leg from the floor and hold for a few breaths. Release and switch sides.

▶ Half locust (*ardha salbhasana*) lifting both legs at the same time, with arms extended and hands beneath the body, palms down.

▶ Half locust (*ardha salbhasana*) lifting both legs at the same time, with arms extended alongside the body, palms down.

▶ Full locust (*salbhasana*) posture both legs extended and lifted from the floor with arms extended, palms down.

▶ Full locust (*salbhasana*) posture both legs extended and lifted from the floor with arms extended past the ears, palms facing each other.

Vinyasa:

▶ Inhale and lift leg(s), exhale and lower leg(s) for several cycles.

Mountain—*Tadasana* (tah-DAHS-anna)/ *Samasthiti* (sa-ma-STI-tee)
tada (mountain) + asana (posture)/*sama* (equal) + *sthiti* (standing still)

Category: Standing

Benefits: Increases body awareness. Balances the nervous system. Cultivates stability, alignment, and equanimity (mental calmness).

Cautions: Knees and hip joints, shoulders if arms are lifted.

Cues to guide students: Stand with feet parallel and hip-width apart. Arms are alongside the body. Ground the feet by lifting and spreading the toes, pressing all four corners of the feet into the floor

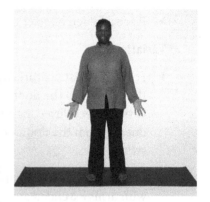

FIGURE 13.28 MOUNTAIN POSE, STANDING VARIATION, FRONT VIEW.

(*samasthiti*). Set the toes back to the floor, keeping the feet active. Engage the core muscles, lengthen the spine, and lift the torso to create space there. Sense the thighs hugging the bones.

Highlight: Leg muscles lifted, shoulders and arms relaxed, spine extended.

Modifications:

▸ Strap or scarf around the thighs and press outward to increase stability.

▸ Block between the thighs and press inward against the block.

▸ Back of heels, sacrum, shoulder blades, or buttocks (gluteal muscles) against the wall. The head is slightly away from the wall.

▸ Supine on the floor, pressing the feet into a wall.

▸ Supine on the floor, pressing the feet into a wall with a block between the thighs.

▸ In a chair, both feet on the floor or some other support such as a block(s) to find 90-degree flexion in the feet, knees, and hips.

Variations:

▸ Bring the feet together, press the legs against each other with the hands in prayer.

▸ Arms overhead—the arms are parallel to each other or in a "V" or "Y" relaxing shoulders away from the ears.

▸ In palm tree (*talasana*), extend the arms overhead and lift the heels off the floor.

Plank/Four-limbed staff—*Phalakasana* (pah-la-KAHS-anna)/*Chaturanga dandasana* (chaht-ah-RON-gah don-DAHS-anna)
phalak (plank) + asana (posture)/*chatur* (four) + *anga* (limb) + *danda* (staff, stick, spinal cord) + asana (posture)

Category: Stabilization

Benefits: Strengthens the core muscles. Aligns the pelvic and shoulder girdles. Cultivates equanimity (mental calmness).

Cautions: Wrist, elbow, neck, shoulder, or back problems. Uncontrolled hypertension.

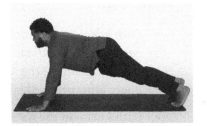

FIGURE 13.29 PLANK POSE, STANDING VARIATION, SIDE VIEW.

Cues to guide students: Start on hands and knees in table (*bharmanasana*) with wrists aligned with shoulders and knees aligned with hips. Press the palms into the floor with fingers spread wide. Release shoulders away from the ears. Press the hands onto the floor and slightly rotate the crease of the elbows in the same direction as the fingers. Engage the core for a neutral lumbar curve. Head, neck, and spine are in natural alignment. Extend one leg and curl the toes under and press

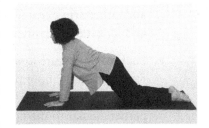

FIGURE 13.30 PLANK POSE, KNEELING VARIATION, SIDE VIEW.

through the heel. To prepare for plank/four-limbed staff (*chaturanga*) or warm up, return knee to floor and extend with the breath. Switch sides and hold for a few breaths. Next, extend one leg at a time, lengthen through both heels, extend spine with neutral alignment, shoulders released away from ears, and press hands into the floor. Engage core muscles and isometrically press legs toward each other and arms toward each other. Hold for several breaths. Release to half plank posture (*ardha chaturanga dandasana*) with knees on the floor or table posture (*bharmanasana*).

Modifications:

▸ In the case of hyperextension, create a micro-bend in your elbows.

▸ Half plank posture (*ardha chaturanga dandasana*) place one knee on the floor, keeping the supporting thigh perpendicular to the mat.

▸ Strap or scarf about upper arms above the elbows.

▸ Block between the thighs.

Variations:

▸ Both knees on the floor for half plank posture (*ardha chaturanga dandasana*) with the forearms on the floor parallel to each other with the palms of the hands lightly pressing into the mat and the upper arms perpendicular to the mat.

▸ Both knees on the floor for half plank posture (*ardha chaturanga dandasana*) with arms extended and palms on the floor.

▸ Half plank posture (*ardha chaturanga dandasana*) with one knee and either arm placement above. Hold for several breaths. Release and repeat on the other leg.

▸ Half plank posture (*ardha chaturanga dandasana*) with the forearms on the floor parallel to each other with the palms of the hands lightly pressing into the mat and the upper arms perpendicular to the floor.

▸ **Knee–chest–chin—*Ashtanga pranam*** (ash-THAN-gah-pra-NAHM)/***Ashtanga namaskara*** (*ashta* [eight] + *anag* [part, limb]) + *namaskara* (bowing, greeting). From plank posture (*phalakasana*) bend the elbows, bring the knees, chest, and chin to the floor, keeping the upper arms hugging the sides of the body.

Vinyasa:

▸ Begin in plank (*phalakasana*), with forearms on the floor, alternate releasing a knee to the floor, moving with the breath.

▸ Begin in plank (*phalakasana*), arms straight (extended), alternate releasing a knee to the floor, moving with the breath.

▸ Begin in plank (*phalakasana*), arms straight (extended), exhaling, flex the elbows and lower the torso to the floor. Inhale returning to plank (*phalakasana*) with straight (extended) arms. Exhaling, bend the elbows and lower the torso toward the mat.

▸ Place the forearms parallel to each other with the palms of the hands lightly pressing into the mat and the upper arms perpendicular to the mat and hold for several breaths.

Seated spinal twist/Half Lord of the Fishes posture—*Ardha matsyendrasana* (are-dah MOT-see-en-DRAHS-asana)
ardha (half) + *matsya* (fish)/Matsyendra (name of a yogi, King of Fish) + asana (posture)

Category: Twist, seated, supine

Benefits: Spinal rotation and flexibility. Calms the nervous system. Supports the diaphragm and intercostal muscles and digestive and excretory systems.

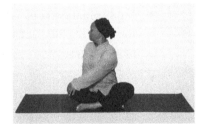

FIGURE 13.31 SEATED SPINAL TWIST POSE, SEATED VARIATION, FRONT VIEW.

Cautions: Lung capacity can be reduced during the twist postures. Back pain, knee, neck problems.

Cues to guide students: Begin in easy seated posture (*sukhasana*) with legs crossed, arms are alongside the body with palms on the floor. Place the sole of the right foot on the floor directly in front of the right hip with toes pointing forward. The right foot crosses the left leg to come to the outside of the left thigh with the right toes pointing forward.

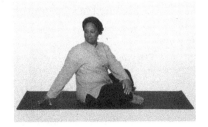

FIGURE 13.32 SEATED SPINAL TWIST POSE, SEATED VARIATION, SIDE VIEW.

Lengthen the spine, interlace the fingers around the shin, engage the core muscles, and ground the sitting bones. Hug the thigh into the torso while isometrically pressing the shin toward the hands. Exhale wrapping the inside of the elbow around the right leg, initiating a twist from the shoulders to the right. Bring the right hand toward the back to rest on the floor near the tailbone (sacrum). Maintaining spinal alignment, gaze over the right shoulder. Hold for several breaths. Return to easy seated posture (*sukhasana*). Notice what sensations are present. Move to the posture on the other side and then notice sensations on that side.

Highlight: Turn from the base of the spine. Head is the last to turn. Breathe fully.

Modifications:

▸ Sit on a wedge, pillow, or folded blanket.

▸ Extend the leg opposite the knee toward the chest.

▸ Hold a strap or scarf behind the back for binding.

Variations:

▸ Wrap the rear arm around the back with the middle finger reaching toward the navel.

▸ Bind spinal twist by reaching the forward arm around and under the bent leg. Reach the other arm behind the back and clasp the hands together.

▸ Supine, arms in a "T," legs crossed at the shins or ankles, move both legs to one side and turn head to the opposite side or in the same direction as the legs.

▸ Supine, arms in a "T," shift hips to one side several inches. Rotate both legs, flex at the knee to one side or with extended legs. Exhale back to center and repeat a few breaths. Then hold for a few breaths. Repeat on the opposite side.

Vinyasa:

▸ Supine, arms in a "T," both knees flexed, exhale and lower both knees to one side turning the head in the opposite direction if desired, inhale back to center, and switch sides with the next breath. Repeat for several rounds. When complete notice sensations that arise.

▸ Seated with hands behind and a few inches away from the torso, fingers pointing away from the body, soles of the feet on the floor wider than hip-width, exhale moving both legs to one side. Inhale turning legs back to center. Exhale legs to the other side. Repeat for several rounds. When complete notice sensations that arise.

Restorative:

▸ Seated with knees flexed and feet on the floor, place a bolster snugly to the side of the left hip, rotate the torso to face the bolster and release the front of the torso to the bolster. Add other props such as a block between the thighs, another bolster to the back or next to a wall as desired. Support the feet with a block or blanket between the feet, under hands, or beneath the head to keep the spine, neck, and head in alignment. Rest here for 5–10 minutes and switch sides.

▸ Supine, arms in a "T," both knees flexed, exhale and lower both knees to one side turning the head in the opposite direction if desired. Use a block, pillow, bolster between or under legs and between or under ankles. Support under neck and shoulders as needed. Adjust space between legs as needed. Rest for 3–5 minutes. Slowly return to center. Notice sensations that arise and when ready repeat on the opposite side.

Staff—*Dandasana* (don-DAHS-anna)
danda (tick, staff) + asana (posture)

Category: Seated, stabilization

Benefits: Improves posture and align-ment. Tones abdominals and thigh mus-cles (quadriceps). Stabilizes the pelvis and shoulders. Lengthens and aligns the spine. Strengthens the quadriceps and stretches the hamstrings.

Cautions: Back, hamstring, and shoulder issues.

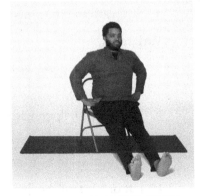

FIGURE 13.33 STAFF POSE, SEATED VARIATION WITH CHAIR, FRONT VIEW.

Cues to guide students: Seated on the floor, extend legs on the floor. Place the palms on the floor alongside the torso. Engage the torso with even hips, neutral pelvis, ground the sitting bones, and lengthen the spine to the crown of the head. Activate the legs by engaging the thighs (quadriceps) and extending through the heels. Inhaling, raise the arms overhead with palms facing inward. Isometrically, press the inner thighs and lower legs together.

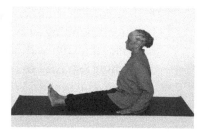

FIGURE 13.34 STAFF POSE, SEATED VARIATION, SIDE VIEW.

Highlight: Rooting/grounding the sitting bones, flex the feet, avoid hyperextending the knees, shoulders down from the ears.

Modifications:

▸ Rolled blanket, bolster, wedge, or pillow beneath the knees.

▸ Back against a wall.

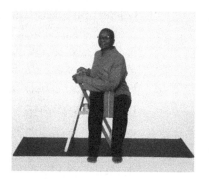

FIGURE 13.35 STAFF POSE, SEATED VARIATION WITH CHAIR AND BLOCKS, FRONT VIEW.

▸ Walk the sitting bones forward and backward.

▸ Block between the thighs.

▸ Block between the hands.

▸ Strap around the thighs pressing out into the strap.

▸ Strap around the arms pressing out into the strap.

Variations:

▸ Lying on the floor, with legs raised with hip flexion with heels on a wall.

▸ Lying on the floor, with legs raised with hip flexion with heels on a wall.

▸ Extend arms to a "Y" position.

▸ Lift one leg off the floor.

▸ Lift both legs off the floor.

Tree—*Vrksasana* (vrik-SHAHS-anna)
vriksa (tree) + asana (posture)

Category: Standing, balance

Benefits: Strengthens legs and feet. Opens and stabilizes the hips.

Cautions: Ankle, knee, or hip issues, particularly knee flexion of the bent knee and hyperextension or pressure on the standing knee.

Cues to guide students: Starting in mountain (*tadasana*) with feet hip-width apart, place the ball of one foot on the floor and externally rotate the leg with the bent knee. Transfer the weight of the body to the standing leg. Lift the ball of the foot from the floor, placing the sole of the foot to the inner thigh of the standing leg with the heel near the groin. Engaging the core muscles, find equal pressure between the foot pressing against the thigh and the thigh pressing against the foot. Reach the arms out to the side to overhead with palms turned inward. Release the shoulders down from the ears.

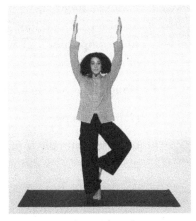

FIGURE 13.36 TREE POSE, STANDING VARIATION, FRONT VIEW.

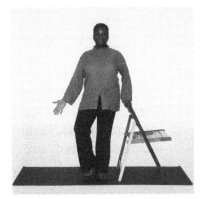

FIGURE 13.37 TREE POSE, STANDING VARIATION WITH CHAIR, FRONT VIEW.

Highlight: Standing leg stability, neutral spine, steady breath.

Modifications:

▸ Stand perpendicular to the wall with bent knee touching the wall for stability.

▸ Place a hand on a chair or the wall for stability. Stand with knee or shin touching a chair or the wall.

▸ One hand on a chair or wall for stability.

▸ Supported by back to wall or front of flexed knee to the wall.

Variations:

▸ Rather than bringing the foot of the bent leg to the inside of the opposite thigh, bring the heel to the opposite ankle with flexed toes on the floor, foot against inner thigh, or outside of the shin to the opposite thigh with hand holding the lower leg—half locust (*ardha salbhasana*).

▸ Hands in prayer (*anjali mudra*) in front of chest.

▸ Hands on hips.

▸ Lift arms laterally to shoulder height, arms overhead to a "V" position or "Y" position.

▸ Lying on the floor with one leg externally rotated, knee flexed, and sole of the foot to the inside of the ankle, shin, or thigh.

Restorative: Find the posture lying on the floor, optionally lying with the side against the wall or sole of foot of the extended leg against the wall. Place a block, blanket, or bolster under the bent knee as needed. Rest here for 5–10 minutes. Notice sensations that arise. Repeat with the other leg.

Triangle—*Utthita trikonasana* (oo-TEE-tah tree-ko-NAHS-anna)

utthita (extended) + *tri* (three) + *kona* (angle) + asana (posture)

Category: Standing, stabilization

Benefits: Strengthens hips, cultivates balance and centering.

Cautions: Neck, hyperextended knees, low back.

Cues to guide students: Starting from warrior 2 (*virabhadrasana* 2), keep the feet grounded. Or begin in a wide stance. Lift the front toes to turn the right foot out 90 degrees. The front heel is aligned with the instep of the back foot. Adjust the width of the stance for preference.

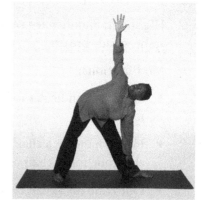

FIGURE 13.38 TRIANGLE POSE, STANDING VARIATION, FRONT VIEW.

Activate both legs and all four corners of the feet. Finding stability, hold for a few breaths with hips squared forward and hands on the waist. Flex front knee over the ankle. The thigh will be parallel to the floor. Placing the left hand on the left hip, raise the right hand to shoulder height and reach out through the right fingertips to the right side. Keeping the hips forward, flex and extend the right knee a few times, then extend the right knee pressing the left hip to the left and the right thigh bone (femur) to the crease of the right hip. Engage the

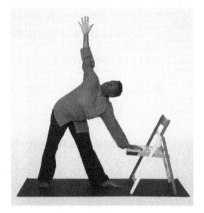

FIGURE 13.39 TRIANGLE POSE, STANDING VARIATION WITH CHAIR, FRONT VIEW.

core muscles. Extending from the left side of the torso and keeping the chest forward, move toward the floor to a place of comfort. Rest the right hand gently on the shin and extend the left hand to the ceiling with the gaze (drishti) forward. Experience several breaths before returning to wide standing or flexing the right knee to return to warrior 2 (*virabhadrasana* 2). Take a few moments to become aware of any sensations that might be present.

Highlight: Strong legs, lengthen the neck, avoid hyperextending knees, and lateral flexion.

Modifications:

▸ Hand on the side of the externally rotated leg on a block, table, the seat of a chair, or the back of a chair.

▸ Hand on the side of the externally rotated leg on a block to the inside or outside of the foot.

▸ Back against a wall.

▸ Reach fingertips of the hand on the side of the externally rotated leg to touch the wall.

Variations:

▸ Gaze (drishti) down at the floor or up at the ceiling.

▸ Top hand behind the back.

- ▸ Hand on the side of the externally rotated leg on the shin or floor to the inside or outside of the foot.

- ▸ Lengthen or shorten the distance of the feet.

- ▸ Variations for the top hand:

  - − Back arm with hand on the waist.

  - − Back arm with forearm behind the back.

  - − Back arm with forearm behind the back with hand on the thigh.

Warrior 1—*Virabhadrasana* 1 (veer-ah-bah-DRAHS-anna)
Virabhadra (the name of a fierce mythical warrior)/*vira* (hero, heroic) + *bhadra* (virtuous, skillful) + asana (posture)

Category: Standing

Benefits: Strengthens legs, flexibility in the hips, and cultivates balance.

Cautions: Misaligned front knee, hyper-extended back knee, impinged shoulders, low back.

Cues to guide students: Beginning in a wide stance with hands on the hips, lift the front toes to turn the right foot out 90 degrees. The front heel is aligned with the instep of the back foot which is turned between 45 and 60 degrees. Adjust the width of the stance for preference. Activate both legs and all four corners of the feet. Square the hips with hands on the

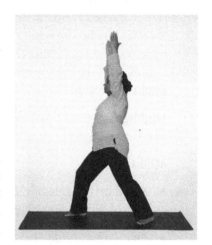

FIGURE 13.40 WARRIOR I POSE, STANDING VARIATION, SIDE VIEW.

waist and flex the front knee over the ankle and the thigh parallel to the floor. Finding stability, hold for a few breaths. Placing the left hand on the left hip, raise the right hand to shoulder height and reach out through the right fingertips to the right side. Keeping the hips forward, flex and extend the right knee a few times, then extend the right knee, pressing the left hip to the left and the right thigh bone (femur) to the crease of the right hip. Engage the core muscles, inhale, and raise the arms out to the side to overhead with palms facing inward. Isometrically, draw the feet toward center. Experience several breaths in the posture before returning to wide standing. Take a few moments to become aware of any sensations that might be present. Repeat on the opposite side.

Highlight: Front knee aligned with heel, hips level, neutral pelvis.

Modifications:

▸ Seated from the side in a chair with the chair supporting the upper body.

▸ One hand on the back of a chair for balance.

▸ Block between the outside of the front knee and a wall.

▸ Block between the front of the knee and a wall.

Variations:

▸ Lengthen or shorten the distance of the feet.

▸ Back heel lifted.

▸ Gaze (drishti) forward.

▸ Back arm with hand on the waist.

▸ Back arm with forearm behind the back.

▸ Bind the back arm behind the back. Front arm extends beneath the front thigh to grasp the hand of the back arm.

▸ Hands in prayer (*anjali mudra*) in front of chest or behind the back.

▸ Hands on hips.

▸ Lift arms laterally to shoulder height, arms overhead to a "V" position or "Y" position.

Vinyasa: Moving with the breath from warrior 1 (*virabhadrasana* 1) hinge forward from the hips, chest toward the thigh, extending arms behind and alongside the body with palms toward the floor.

Warrior 2—*Virabhadrasana 2* (veer-ah-bah-DRAHS-anna)
Virabhadra (the name of a fierce mythical warrior)/*vira* (hero, heroic) + *bhadra* (virtuous, skillful) + asana (posture)

Category: Standing

Benefits: Strengthens legs and feet. Tones pelvic floor and reproductive and urinary systems. Improves circulation to the extremities.

Cautions: Misaligned front knee, hyperextended back knee, impinged shoulders, low back.

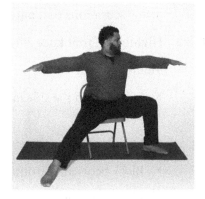

FIGURE 13.41 WARRIOR 2 POSE, SEATED VARIATION WITH CHAIR, FRONT VIEW.

Cues to guide students: Starting from a wide stance, lift the front toes to turn the right foot out 90 degrees. The front heel is aligned with the instep of the back foot. Adjust the width of the stance for preference. Activate both legs and all four corners of the feet. Finding stability, hold for a few breaths with hips squared forward and hands on the waist. Flex front knee over the ankle. The thigh will be parallel to the floor. Keeping the hips forward, flex and extend the right knee a few times, then flex the right knee and draw the right thigh bone (femur) to the crease of the right hip. Engage the core muscles and lengthen the spine, keeping the chest forward. Experience several breaths before returning to wide standing.

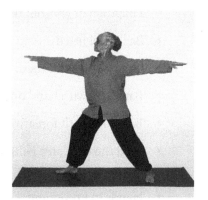

FIGURE 13.42 WARRIOR 2 POSE, STANDING VARIATION, FRONT VIEW.

Take a few moments to become aware of any sensations that might be present. Repeat on the opposite side.

Highlight: Front knee aligned with heel, hips level, neutral pelvis, shoulders down.

Modifications:

▸ Seated in a chair with the chair supporting the upper body.

▸ One hand on the back of a chair for balance.

▸ Block between the outside of the front knee and a wall.

▸ Block between the front of the knee and a wall.

▸ Back of the body on the wall.

Variations:

▸ Lengthen or shorten the distance of the feet.

▸ Gaze (drishti) forward or on the middle finger of the front hand.

▸ Back arm with hand on the waist.

▸ Back arm with forearm behind the back.

▸ Hands in prayer (*anjali mudra*) in front of chest or behind the back.

▸ Hands on hips.

▸ Lift front hand to the ceiling and release back arm to the outside of the back thigh. Inhale allowing the back arm to move down the leg toward the floor, **reverse warrior—*viparita virabhadrasana*** (vip-par-ee-tah veer-ar-bah-DRAHS-anna) *viparita* (reverse) + *Virabhadra* (the name of a fierce mythical warrior)/*vira* (hero, heroic) + *bhadra* (virtuous, skillful) + asana (posture).

Vinyasa:

▸ Moving with the breath straighten the front leg and bring the arms overhead. Exhale and return to warrior 2 (*virabhadrasana* 2). Repeat several full breaths.

▸ Moving with the breath straighten the front leg, rotate the front foot forward, and bring the arms overhead. Exhale and return to warrior 2 (*virabhadrasana* 2). Repeat several full breaths.

CHAPTER 14

How to Teach Hand Gestures (Mudras)

Practicing mudras can take place in a quiet and private place or discreetly anywhere.

The Sanskrit word for hand gestures is mudra. Mudras are sometimes called "seals" or "locks," and are also combinations of postures (asana), breathing (pranayama), and locks (bandha).[1] They are a nonverbal method that communicates moods, intentions, and attitudes.[2] Gestures can also consciously bring about psychological or spiritual attitudes. For the purpose of this text mudras will be specific to hand gestures. Also, cues will in some cases describe actions for one hand, so duplicate the gesture for the other hand unless identified otherwise.

Hand gestures have been a part of the indigenous cultures of Africa, Fiji, Egypt, Rome, Greece, India, China, Australia, Inuit, and North America for thousands of years.[3] Some hand gestures are universal, such as clapping hands of joy, a hand over the heart for love or sympathy, or the pointed index finger moving left and right or in a circle (Italy, Japan, and Indigenous peoples of America's culture) to indicate no. Gestures are also part of some spiritual practices such as palms together in prayer (*anjali mudra*). Plato identified hand gestures in Greece in categories for comedy, tragedy, and satire. Romans even held best hand gesture dancer competitions. Some Indigenous peoples of America communicated with hand sign communication in front of strangers and later played a role in communicating with hearing-impaired children. Western cultures now use hand gestures mostly as communication gestures.

Hand gestures (mudras) can be practiced alone or in combination with postures (asana), breathing practices (pranayama), or locks (bandhas).

Joseph and Lillian LePage explain that there are numerous sensory and motor nerve endings in the fingers, making the fingers "a powerful vehicle for communicating directly with the brain and the rest of the body."[4]

Mudras can be selected for specific purposes. Hand gestures also support hand health and can be beneficial in treating arthritis of the hands with regular practice. Core qualities are associated with mudras as they unlock energetic keys. While mudras are not magic bullets that help with health conditions, their core characteristics are helpful for unfolding positive qualities along the path to health and healing.

Practicing mudras can take place in a quiet and private place or discreetly anywhere. They can also be part of a pranayama or asana practice. The hand can be included in different formations during movement or while seated comfortably. Work up to holding the mudra position for 5 minutes using just enough pressure to notice a flow of energy.

There are numerous mudras to include in the practice, but for a start consider the following six hand gestures: *anjali mudra, dhyana mudra, gyan mudra, padma mudra, shunya mudra,* and *vaikhara mudra.*

Anjali mudra (ahn-JALEE moo-DRAH)
anjali (reverence) + mudra (gesture)

Purpose: Invoking divine union. *Anjali mudra* is sometimes called prayer position and used when saying *Namaste.* This is a powerful gesture of gratitude and a symbol of thanks and seeing the holy light in self and in others. The gesture directs breath and awareness to the center of the chest and supports turning focus inward. It is also used as a greeting and a way of communicating recognition of unity.

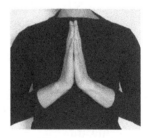

FIGURE 14.1 ANJALI MUDRA, FRONT VIEW.

Cautions: None

Cues for guiding students: Bring your palms together at your heart center with your fingers pointing upward.

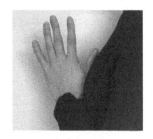

FIGURE 14.2 ANJALI MUDRA, SIDE VIEW.

Dhyana mudra (dee-YANA moo-DRAH)/
Jnana mudra (YA-na moo-DRAH)
dhyana (meditation)/jnana (wisdom) + mudra (gesture)

Purpose: Awakening clear seeing. The gesture is believed to invoke a sense of increased focus and concentration and is a good gesture for sitting in quiet contemplation or meditation. This mudra represents total balance.

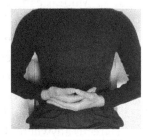

FIGURE 14.3 DHYANA MUDRA, FRONT VIEW.

Cautions: None

Cues for guiding students: Place the back of the left hand in the lap with the back of the right hand resting in the palm of the left hand. Bring the tips of the thumbs together to complete a circle.

Gyan mudra (GUY-yon moo-DRAH)/
Chin mudra (chin moo-DRAH)
gyan (knowledge, wisdom)/chin (consciousness) + mudra (gesture)

Purpose: Surrender to the divine. It is a common mudra used in yoga and meditation practices and is believed to cultivate silence in the mind. The gesture also helps with full diaphragmatic breathing by expanding the breath and awareness the front of the torso. The exhalation is gently extended allowing a sense of balance and harmony to move inward.

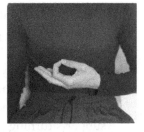

FIGURE 14.4 GYAN MUDRA, FRONT VIEW.

Cautions: None

Cues for guiding students: With the palms turned upward on the thighs or knees, the tips of the thumbs touch the tips of the index fingers. Remaining fingers are straight and relaxed.

Padma mudra (pod-MAH moo-DRAH)
padma (lotus) + mudra (gesture)

Purpose: Unconditional love. This gesture is also called lotus mudra. It is believed to evoke compassion and loving-kindness and represents positive transformation. The gesture directs breath and awareness into the chest to instill a sense of lightness and openness. Imagine the layers of mud fall away until the true nature emerges.

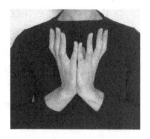

FIGURE 14.5 PADMA MUDRA, FRONT VIEW.

Cautions: Arthritis in hands, stenosing tenosynovitis (trigger finger), or other hand and finger conditions. Wrist, finger, or palm surgery.

Cues for guiding students: Bring your palms together at your heart center with your fingers pointing upward. Keep the thumbs and last fingers together. Extend the other six fingers open and apart pointing upward. Imagine hands forming a lotus blossom at heart center.

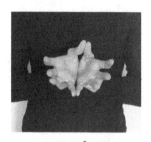

FIGURE 14.6 PADMA MUDRA, TOP VIEW.

Shunya mudra (shewn-YA moo-DRAH)
shunya (zero, empty) + mudra (gesture)

Purpose: Opening to transformation. Also called *shuni mudra*, it is considered to foster the ability to be patient and disciplined and helps to cultivate new ways of seeing. The breath and awareness are directed to the throat and neck area and help to release throat and neck tension.

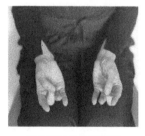

FIGURE 14.7 SHUNYA MUDRA, FRONT VIEW.

Cautions: Arthritis in hands, stenosing tenosynovitis (trigger finger), or other hand and finger conditions.

Cues for guiding students: Bring the tip of the middle finger to the base of the palm. Press the thumb gently against the middle finger below the knuckle. Allow the other fingers to remain relaxed and straight. Rest the hand on the thigh or knee.

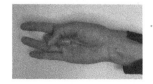

FIGURE 14.8 SHUNYA MUDRA, TOP VIEW.

Vaikhara mudra (vaee-KA-ra moo-DRAH)
vaikhara (solid, protective) + *mudra* (gesture)

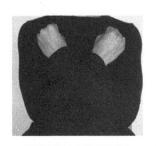

FIGURE 14.9 VAIKHARA MUDRA, FRONT VIEW.

Purpose: Gesture of the protective shield. Fosters a sense of empowerment and enhances alertness. With this gesture, the awareness, breath, and energy are directed into the chest. The thymus gland is located behind the upper sternum. This gland supports immune system health and starts to shrink (atrophy) into adulthood. As alertness increases, awareness of the environment increases including the five elements of nature (earth, water, fire, air, and space). Relaxes upper back muscles.

Cautions: Arthritis in hands, stenosing tenosynovitis (trigger finger), or other hand and finger conditions.

Cues for guiding students: Make fists with both hands with thumbs across the second joint of the ring fingers. Cross the inside of the right fist across the chest to rest on the left side of the chest below the shoulder joint. Cross the left forearm over the right forearm to rest the left fist on the right side of the chest below the shoulder joint. Soften the shoulders and maintain natural spinal alignment.

CHAPTER 15

Meditation as a Healing Practice

May you know that love is your sacred birthright, that you are loved and held by transcendent and ancestral powers that see you beyond appearances and circumstances, that love you even when you are not loving yourself. (Shelly Harrell, PhD, The Soulfulness Center, with permission)

Recalling the eight limbs of yoga, postures (asana) and breath control (pranayama) prepare the practitioner for experiencing two other limbs. Meditation is a path the practitioner uses to access and experience drawing the senses inward through releasing external distractions (pratyahara), concentration (dharana), and meditation (dhyana).

Meditation has long-term effects with long-term meditators experiencing less heart disease and cancer than non-meditators. Those with insomnia sleep better and some experience reduced chronic pain.[1] The brain is directly affected by meditation, and thus the rest of the body. According to Rebecca Gladding, MD, the ventromedial prefrontal cortex, which runs things through a "me" lens, activates after the first few minutes.[2] After starting to focus the lateral prefrontal cortex activates and overrides the "me" thoughts for a more rational and balanced position. In other words, the "me" center of the brain quiets. After 8–12 weeks of daily meditation, the dorsomedial prefrontal cortex, the part of the brain that helps develop empathy, is activated.

Gail Parker, PhD, explains in her book *Restorative Yoga for Ethnic and Race-Based Stress and Trauma* that meditation facilitates clarity of thought.[3] When meditating, the meditator cultivates awareness of their inner world that leads to clarity, and through self-study cultivates higher levels of consciousness. Those who meditate regularly experience less anxiety and stress.

As an only child, Shelly Harrell, PhD, cultivated practices early in life that evolved into contemplative and meditation practices. She has participated in meditation and contemplative practices for most of her life.[4] Harrell, having taught meditation in various settings, stated that her "sensibilities around meditation are tied closely to [her] own diasporic African and African American cultural influences." She founded the Soulfulness Center to cultivate meaningful practices for transformative change. A sample of her work can be found in the following two loving-kindness meditations that may resonate in the Black community.

MAY YOU BE FREE

MAY YOU BE SAFE AND PROTECTED
May you be safe from dangers and harm. May you know your soul's refuge, that inner sanctuary untouched by circumstances.

MAY YOU BE WELL
May you have relief from any ailments and be as healthy and strong as possible. May you bring attention and care to the health of your body, mind, heart, and soul.

MAY YOU LOVE AND BE LOVED
May love and compassion warm your heart and soothe your soul. May you see through the eyes of love, listen with the ears of love, and act from a place of love.

MAY YOU BE AT PEACE
May you find your calm center within the storms of life, living with ease and grace. May you find that place of quietude, stillness, and deep serenity within your soul.

MAY YOU BE HAPPY
May you experience awe and beauty and celebrations and laughter. May you feel your joyful, soulful aliveness and may your soul smile with inner contentment.

MAY YOU BE FREE
May you experience the emancipation of your mind, the opening of your heart, and the illumination of your soul. May you be free to express your truth and be your authentic self, free to

*pursue your purpose, share your gifts, and manifest your highest
calling for your life, the lives of others, and the world.
May peace and love wash over you—replenishing,
refreshing, and nourishing your soul.
May you be safe and protected.
May you be well.
May you love and be loved.
May you be at peace.
May you be happy.
May you be free.*

Shelly Harrell, PhD
The Soulfulness Center
with permission

YOU ARE LOVED

*May peace and love wash over you, replenishing,
refreshing and nourishing your soul.
May you love and be loved.
May you open yourself to fully receive love, allowing love to pour
into your being, to warm your heart and soothe your soul.
May you see through the eyes of love, listen with the
ears of love, and act from the ground of love.
May you bring love, compassion, patience, and forgiveness to
yourself, a loving voice of care to the tender places within.
May you treat yourself and others with kindness, honoring
the vulnerabilities of our shared human journey.
May you know that love is your sacred birthright, that you
are loved and held by transcendent and ancestral powers
that see you beyond appearances and circumstances, that
love you even when you are not loving yourself.
May you celebrate the eternal, restorative, and transformative
power of love to heal, uplift, liberate, connect, and save us all.
You are loved.*

Shelly Harrell, PhD
The Soulfulness Center
with permission

Meditation, mindfulness, and contemplative practices move the practitioner from analysis to wisdom and insight. Contemplative and restorative practices are also the bedrock of the Black Yoga Teachers Alliance (BYTA). BYTA's flagship program, Yoga as a Peace Practice (YPP)™, is a post-lineage program that facilitates the contemplative aspects of yoga to address the trauma of violence experienced in modern society.[5] The training cultivates "resilience, inner peace, and well-being in individuals, families, and communities." It also prepares yoga teachers to "offer yoga that can be practiced beyond the yoga mat and brought into everyday life."

Both Harrell and BYTA resonate with The Tree of Contemplative Practices created by The Center for Contemplative Mind in Society.[6] The tree has its roots in awareness, communion, and connection. The branches of the tree indicate active, creative, generative, relational, movement, stillness, and ritual/cyclical ways to practice contemplatively.

For those students that think that they cannot meditate, Roger Walsh, MD, PhD, suggests a variety of ways to meditate such as single tasking, focused breathing, or centering.[7] Single tasking is the act of focusing on a task. It could be walking, drinking a cup of tea, *shinrin-yoku* (forest bathing), washing the dishes, observing the ocean, listening to music, or journaling. Focused breathing can include any of the breathing practices discussed in this book, among others. Centering can include contemplative reading, inquiry, and interoceptive awareness (e.g., noticing an itch or an emotion and the sensations associated with it). Another option is *yoga nidra*, yogic sleep.

Yoga nidra

It is the art of non-doing.

Yoga nidra (yoga of sleep) is a practice composed of a series of breath, body, and awareness techniques that leads to a state of non-doing. It is the art of non-doing. It is an ancient regenerative and transformational practice described in the Upanishads, a text that describes the nature of the universe and self-realization. Swami Satyananda Saraswati stated that *yoga nidra* is a technique for learning to consciously relax and to truly relax; the experience surpasses sleep and *doing* something to relax.[8] *Yoga nidra* is the state of non-doing that allows access to changes in dream states, deep sleep, and the state beyond. Sometimes it is referred to as "deep relaxation with inner awareness." It is an experience of turning inward.

Yoga nidra is a deep form of meditation that can be practiced for numerous reasons, such as to reduce stress or to address insomnia, anxiety, or fear. In his book *Yoga Nidra: The iRest Meditative Practice for Deep Relaxation and Healing*, Richard Miller, PhD, explains that the practice of *yoga nidra* as brought to us through ancient teachings is beyond expression, yet an experientially heartfelt presence that is interconnected with all life. It is a realization that brings the *"peace that passeth all understanding."*[9] Tracee Stanley, author of *Radiant Rest: Yoga Nidra for Deep Relaxation and Awakened Clarity*, describes *yoga nidra* as a powerful practice that "transcends our ability to truly describe."[10]

Yoga nidra is a form of meditation in which the practitioner experiences brainwave states similar to sleep. When in this state, the practitioner can be less engaged with thoughts and becomes more of an observer of thoughts. The practice begins with body, breath, and awareness techniques that guide the practitioner to a state of resting in awareness, not practicing being aware, but in a state of non-doing. According to Kamini Desai, PhD, author of *Yoga Nidra: The Art of Trans-formational Sleep*, *yoga nidra* has substantial possibility and yet is "one of the…most under-appreciated practices of Yoga."[11] See the Resources section of this book for a list of several sources of additional information about *yoga nidra*.

Glossary

The glossary provides an explanation of the general use of the terms. For a more formal definition, please consult a standard collegiate dictionary.

Abhyasa The discipline of committed spiritual practice in yoga.

Aboriginal A population of people considered native to a geographic area.

Acculturation Changes to one people's culture by another, usually by domination or force.

Adherence Following an instruction or protocol with fidelity.

Agonist A muscle that causes contraction or that shortens a muscle.

Ahimsa A yoga attribute of the yama yogic principle: abstaining from all forms of violence, physical or emotional.

Allostatic load A measurement of the physiological dysregulation caused by chronic stress on the body.

Anatomy The study of the physical body structures and their functions.

Ancestor Member of a family's lineage.

Antagonist The opposing muscle to the agonist, to either lengthen or shorten a muscle back to its original position.

Aparigraha A yoga attribute of the yama yogic principle: valuing others' gifts and talents in the absence of envy or jealousy.

Appropriation To take possession of without consent.

Asana The physical practice of hatha yoga that includes specific postures that provide beneficial physical and energetic alignment for the human body and mind.

Ashtanga The systematic yoga practice codified by Patanjali in the Yoga Sutras that includes eight primary practices ("eight limbs") as a way of life toward purification of the mind, body, and soul. The eight limbs are: yama, niyama, asana, pranayama, pratyahara, dharana, dhyana, and samadhi.

Asteva A yoga attribute of the yama yogic principle: honoring the gifts of others by not coveting (desiring) what is not one's own.

Avidya A state of spiritual ignorance that keeps the seeker from understanding the true Self.

Ayurveda The Indian science of medicine.

Bandhas Energy locks or "seals" that are practiced to direct the flow of prana (energy) through four major channels of the body: *mula bandha* (the "root" energy lock located in the pelvic floor), *uddiyana bandha* (the "upward rising" energy lock located in the abdominal region), *jalandhara bandha* (the "chin" energy lock located in the throat region), and *maha bandha* (the "triple lock" that supports the opening and flow of the three lower bandhas).

Bhakti The yoga practice of devotion.

BIPOC An acronym for Black, Indigenous, People of Color.

Brahmacharya A yoga attribute of the yama yogic principle: being patient and empathetic toward self and others.

Characteristic An attribute assigned to describe a specific quality of a person or condition.

Chronic A condition that occurs consistently for a long period of time.

Codify To organize a process systematically.

Community A group of people joined together by like interests, culture, or familiar characteristics.

Consciousness The state of awareness of the mind and one's own existence.

Contraction The process of making smaller. In anatomy, contraction of a muscle makes it smaller than its actual length.

Contraindication A specific reason that certain actions, procedures, or activities should not be taken due to prescribed health conditions.

Critical race theory (CRT) The study of the historical impact of the dominant culture's social, political, legal, economic, and religious norms on racial equity and how this shapes our worldview.

Cues Verbal prompts of instruction to assist yoga students' understanding of how to practice yoga.

Culture An established set of principles, practices, and beliefs that are embraced by a group of people as a way of life.

Dharana The practice of concentrated effort of the mind. One of the eight limbs of ashtanga yoga.

Dharma The principle of living in accordance with one's true nature or purpose and fulfilling one's duties and responsibilities in life. According to yoga philosophy, living a life of dharma requires self-awareness, self-discipline, and a commitment to doing what is right.

Dhyana The practice of meditation. One of the eight limbs of ashtanga yoga.

Diaphragmatic breathing Abdominal or "belly" breathing through the optimal use of the lower diaphragm during inhalation and exhalation. In diaphragmatic breathing, the abdominal diaphragm descends on inhalation to encourage the full extension of the lungs. On exhalation, the abdominal diaphragm ascends (lifts) upward to support the expulsion of air out of the lungs.

Diaspora The dispersion of a people living outside of their homeland of origin.

Dinacharya A systematic daily routine established in the science of ayurveda to promote health and well-being. The ayurvedic daily routine consists of cleansing, massage, exercise, study, meditation, and yoga.

Discernment The practice of distinguishing thoughts, concepts, and beliefs objectively.

Disproportionate Unequal; inequalities usually associated with socio-economic and health and other societal systems.

Dosha The constitutional qualities of human life that are composed of the universal elements of earth, water, air, ether, and fire. In ayurveda medicine, the doshas provide keys to diagnosing unbalances in health. The doshas consist of three main energetic types; however, combinations of the three may be present in people. The three main doshas and their primary elements are vata (air and ether), pitta (fire and water), and khapha (earth and water).

Drishti The practice of establishing a meditative state through focused gaze.

Dysregulation An imbalance or impairment to a physical, metabolic, or psychological process.

Efficacy A measure of effectiveness in its most pure form.

Eight limbs of yoga A systematic practice that supports overall healing and well-being. In the Yoga Sutras of Patanjali (2.28) practicing the eight limbs of yoga removes impurities and obstacles that hinder spiritual and moral growth and development.

Energetic The vibrant action of body, mind, and spirit; vitality.

Enslavement Unlawful subjugation of human beings against their will.

Epidemiology The study and analysis of disease within a population.

Evidence-based A strategy agreed upon to support a specific action such as health promotion based on a series of objective observations that provide evidence for employing such action.

Exhalation The process of expelling breath or air out of the lungs.

Explicit bias The overt practice of prejudice or racism.

Extension A physiological term for increasing the angle between two body parts.

Extrinsic External; not an essential part of a process or thing.

Faith Belief or knowing based on one's intuition or deep sense of consciousness.

Fascia Connective tissue that binds to muscles and all other organ systems.

Flexion A physiological term for decreasing the angle between two body parts.

Foundation The base of a structure that provides stability.

Guna Three fundamental qualities of nature. The three qualities are *sattva* (purity, lightness, and harmony), *rajas* (activity, restlessness, and passion), and *tamas* (inertia, darkness, and ignorance). The *gunas* influence our physical, mental, and emotional states. As we navigate these states and can cultivate *sattva*, a state of balance and harmony can be achieved.

Guru Master teacher of yoga.

Hatha The physical practice of yoga that includes the practice of asanas. In Sanskrit, *ha* (sun) and *tha* (moon) define this practice as one that balances the qualities of these two energies.

Healing Our innate processes for rejuvenating body, mind, and spirit.

Health benefits Scientific researched-based processes and actions a person takes to enhance their quality of life.

Health care The individual responsibility and actions taken for maintaining one's health and well-being.

Healthcare An established industry or system designed to support the well-being of a community.

Health disparity Differences in health-promoting treatments that cause an unequal status of well-being among varying people within a population.

Health equity An environment in which everyone has the opportunity to achieve their highest level of health.

Health literacy A comprehensive understanding of various health conditions.

Heritage The legacy of a people that includes their birthright.

History The chronological life journey of mankind, written and/or oral.

Hoodoo A spiritual practice that includes rituals (such as incantations and sacrificing) and the use of herbal remedies to influence physical, mental, and emotional healing.

Human The manifestation of nature in a superior form of life whose characteristics are intellectually and morally in tune with the laws of creation.

Implicit bias Unaware practice of prejudice or racism.

Indigenous Native in origin.

Inhalation The process of absorbing breath or air into the lungs.

Inquiry Investigative questioning.

Intercostal The muscles of the ribcage.

Intersectionality A political framework that defines how the social, economic, health, race, and gender identity societal constructs impact systemic discrimination and privilege.

Intrinsic Internal; an essential part of a process or thing.

Inversion Reverse in position. In an asana practice, the physical positioning of the head placement being lower than the hips.

Ishvara pranidhana A yoga attribute of the niyama yogic principle: surrender to the source of Life through the practice of worshipping God.

Kemetic yoga A system of spiritual self-development based on ancient Egyptian philosophy.

Kirtan The Buddhist and yoga practice of chanting or singing in praise of the Divine.

Kosha A layer of energy. In Sanskrit, Kosha translates as "sheath," the "sheath covering for a saber/sword." The Yoga Sutras describes five sheaths—*panca maya kosha*—that are layered upon themselves and thus somewhat interconnected. The five *panca maya koshas* are: anamaya, pranamaya, manomaya, vijanamaya, and anandamaya.

Kundalini An essential source of energy that lies dormant within us. Located in the base of the spine, the practice of yoga cultivates the awakening of this energy as a means of purification and obtaining higher states of consciousness.

Lateral In physiology, a side bending position of the body.

Life expectancy A scientific calculation of the term of a population's life based on lifestyle and other environmental factors.

Lineage The succession of a culture's historical knowledge passed from teacher to pupil/disciple.

Mantra The recitation of specific thoughts or phrases practiced to cultivate one-pointed focused concentration and feelings of bliss.

Marginalization Attitudes and actions within the dominant culture that negatively impact the overall quality of life for certain segments of society, especially people of color, the economically disadvantaged, and members of the LGBTQIA communities.

Meditation The practice of objective observation of one's consciousness. One of the eight limbs of yoga.

Metabolism The biological processes of the human body that use energy to support healthy functioning of our organ systems.

Mitigate To stop or control something undesirable.

Modification Enhancing the standard way of practicing a yoga asana (posture) to make it more accessible for practitioners, often through the use of props such as chairs, yoga blocks, straps, blankets, and/or bolsters.

Morbidity An unhealthy state due to the impact of disease accumulated through lifestyle and environment factors.

Mortality Conditions that lead to the rate of death in a society.

Mudra The Sanskrit word for hand gestures. Mudras are sometimes called "seals" or "locks," and are also combinations of postures (asana), breathing (pranayama), and locks (bandha). They are a non-verbal method that communicates moods, intentions, and attitudes. Gestures can also consciously bring about psychological or spiritual attitudes.

Nature The intrinsic composition of elements that make up the earth and all its inhabitants.

Nidra In Sanskrit, Nidra is translated as "sleep." The practice of *yoga nidra* is a systematic approach to cultivating total rest and relaxation—physically, mentally, and emotionally.

Niyama The yogic principle of introspection or observance that includes *saucha, santosha, tapas, svadhyaya,* and *ishvara pranidhana.*

Nonadherence Failure to follow a prescribed protocol to support a specific health condition.

Oppression A systematic process of abuse through the denial of basic human rights.

Oral tradition The verbal transmission of wisdom, knowledge, and rituals of a culture shared and maintained as historical record.

Pain Physical, mental, and emotional sensations of discomfort caused by trauma.

Parasympathetic nervous system The portion of the autonomic nervous system that supports rest and relaxation.

Patanjali The 2nd-century South Asian sage acknowledged as the "Father of Yoga." Patanjali formally developed and codify a systemic process for acquiring spiritual wisdom through self-realization: ashtanga, the eight limbs of yoga.

Pathologic A pattern of disorder that leads to disease.

People of global majority A political term to define races of people that are not recognized as members of the world dominant culture.

Perspective A point of view based on one's contextual understanding of the subject at hand.

Philosophy The study of the laws of nature using logical reasoning.

Physiology The science of the physical processes of the human body's organ systems.

Practitioner A person who actively participates in a specific endeavor.

Prakriti In the science of ayurveda, the human constitution and nature.

Pranayama A compound term that means vital life force (prana) and control (yama) or expansion (ayama). It is a series of practices that supports the control and expansion of the breath to increase vitality and calm the mind. One of the eight limbs of ashtanga yoga.

Pratyahara The practice of introspection without the distraction of sensory stimuli. One of the eight limbs of ashtanga yoga.

Primer An introductory text that provides the basic elements of a subject.

Prone A reclining position face down (on one's stomach).

Psychosocial The influence of social lifestyle factors on emotional development.

Racism A system of structuring opportunity and assigning value based on the social interpretation of how one looks (what we call "race"), that unfairly disadvantages some individuals and communities, and unfairly advantages some individuals and communities.

Research-based A systematic process that is developed and implemented through scientific study that includes a standard protocol to assure its validity.

Resilience The ability to thrive against opposition.

Restorative Practices that replenish the health and well-being of one's body, mind, and spirit.

Retention To hold or maintain in a steady state.

Ritual An act within a culture that is considered significant to the foundation of their spiritual beliefs and practices.

Sage A person revered for their spiritual wisdom.

Samadhi The state of bliss acquired through the practice of ashtanga yoga. One of the eight limbs of ashtanga yoga.

Santosha A yoga attribute of the niyama yogic principle: contentment of mind in the absence of desire.

Satya A yoga attribute of the yama yogic principle: speaking the truth regardless of the circumstance.

Saucha A yoga attribute of the niyama yogic principle: observances and practices for purification of the body, mind, and emotions.

Segregation The practice of separation based on discriminative factors such as race, gender, and/or religious beliefs.

Self-care Taking personal responsibility for one's health and well-being.

Social construct An accepted set of ideas based on a society's perception.

Social determinants of health (SDOH) Factors that influence the state of health and well-being. Factors may include: living environment, economic, education, food access, race, ethnicity, and gender.

Socioeconomic status The social stature of a person or group of people based on their education, occupation, and earning ability.

Sojourn Residing outside of one's home for a period of time.

Somatic Physical movement of the body.

Stress The physiological response to perceive threat or trauma.

Structural racism The perpetuation of racial discrimination within a society upheld throughout all of its systems: education, health, economic, housing, and justice.

Student A person in pursuit of knowledge.

Supine A reclining position face up (on one's back).

Sutra A written verse in the Yoga Sutras of Patanjali. The transliteration of sutra means "thread."

Svadhyaya A yoga attribute of the niyama yogic principle: the commitment to cultivate one's journey as a lifelong learner.

Sympathetic nervous system The portion of the autonomic nervous system that activates the fight or flight response.

Systematic racism Racial discrimination practices that are established throughout a society's institutions.

Tapas A yoga attribute of the niyama yogic principle: acceptance of life's inevitable challenges and limitations as potential areas of growth to gain wisdom.

Telomere DNA structures at the end of chromosomes; they are markers for aging.

Trauma An injury, physical or perceived, caused by force.

Ujjayi The yoga pranayama practice that supports the anatomical alignment of breathing utilizing the lungs, diaphragm inhalation and exhalation.

Variation Changing the standard postural form for practicing a specific yoga asana/posture.

Vinyasa A hatha yoga practice of continuous movements between asanas (postures).

Vodun A religious practice originating in West Africa based on oral tradition and preserved through rituals of song and dance. Practitioners of the faith are initiated through various acts of worship.

Yama The yogic principle of abstinence that include: *ahimsa, satya, asteya, brahmacharya*, and *aparigraha*.

Yang The strong, dynamic force of energy; often considered "masculine" energy.

Yin The subtle, nurturing force of energy; often considered "feminine" energy.

Yoga In Sanskrit, yoga is translated as "yoking, joining or union." The philosophic practice of personal inquiry that leads to deeper understanding of the Divine or Ultimate Creator of life.

Resources

The resources listed here include books, periodicals, and websites that the authors found useful in their own yoga journeys. We offer them as a starting place for further personal education and inquiry. The list provides a variety of perspectives and should stimulate your curiosity.

ADAPTABLE/ACCESSIBLE YOGA

Bondy, D. (2019) *Yoga for Everyone: 50 Poses for Every Type of Body*. Penguin Random House.

Danzig, M. T. (2018) *Yoga for Amputees: The Essential Guide to Finding Wholeness after Limb Loss for Yoga Students and Their Teachers*. Sacred Oak Publishing.

Eisenberg, M. (2015) *Adaptive Yoga Moves Any Body*. Orange Cat Press.

Grilley, P. (2012) *Yin Yoga: Principles and Practice*. White Cloud Press.

Krentzman, R. (2016) *Yoga for a Healthy Back: A Teacher's Guide to Spinal Health through Yoga Therapy*. Singing Dragon.

Moonaz, S. & Byron, E. (2019) *Yoga Therapy for Arthritis: A Whole Person Approach to Movement and Lifestyle*. Singing Dragon.

Peterson, M. (2011) *Move without Pain*. Sterling.

Saraswati, S. W. (1984) *Yoga and Cardiovascular Management*. Yoga Publications Trust.

Shapiro, D. (2006) *Your Body Speaks Your Mind*. Sounds True.

AFRICAN DIASPORA/BLACK HISTORY

Ashby, M. (2005) *Egyptian Yoga: The Philosophy of Enlightenment*. 10th Ed. Cruzian Mystic Books.

Ashby, M. (2005) *The African Origins: African Origins of African Civilization, Mystic Religion, Yoga Mystical*. Cruzian Mystic Books.

Black Yoga Teachers Alliance www.blackyogateachersalliance.org.

Brewster, F. (2020) *The Racial Complex: A Jungian Perspective on Culture and Race*. Routledge.

Brewster, F. (2019) *Archetypal Grief: Slavery's Legacy of Intergenerational Child Loss*. Routledge.

Brewster, F. & Morgan, H. (2022) *Racial Legacies: Jung, Politics and Culture*. Routledge.

Bynum, E. B. (2021) *Our African Unconscious: The Black Origins of Mysticism and Psychology*. Inner Traditions Audio.

Coleman, M. C. (2023) *We Heal Together: Rituals and Practices for Building Community and Connection*. Shambhala Publications.

Drake, St. C. & Cayton, J. R. (1945/2015) *Black Metropolis: A Study of Negro Life in a Northern City.* University of Chicago Press.

Evans, S. Y. (2021) *Black Women's Yoga History: Memoirs of Inner Peace.* SUNY Press.

Hafiz, S. (2018) *The Healing: One Woman's Journey from Poverty to Inner Riches.* Parallax Press.

Hunter, F. (2021) *Spiritually Fly: Wisdom, Meditation and Yoga to Elevate Your Soul.* Sounds True.

Long, J. (2016) *The Uncommon Yogi: A History of Blacks and Yoga in the US.* www.youtube.com/watch?v=xQqSdB9PD38.

Mitchell, S. (2018) *Sacred Instructions: Indigenous Wisdom for Living Spirit-Based Change.* North Atlantic Books.

Mydral, G. (2017) *An American Dilemma: The Negro Problem and Modern Democracy*, Vol. 1. Black and African American Studies. Routledge.

Some, M. P. (1999) *The Healing Wisdom of Africa: Finding Life Purpose through Nature, Ritual, and Community.* Jeremy P. Tarcher/Putnam.

Williams, A. K. (2002) *Being Black: Zen and the Art of Living Fearlessness and Grace.* Penguin Books.

Williams, A. K., Owens, L. R., & Syedullah, J. (2016) *Radical Dharma: Talking Race, Love, and Liberation.* North Atlantic Books.

Yetunde, P. A. (2020) *Black and Buddhist: What Buddhism Can Teach Us about Race, Resilience, Transformation, and Freedom.* Shambhala.

ANATOMY

Farhi, D. & Stuart, L. (2017) *Pathways to a Centered Body.* Embodied Wisdom Publishing.

Kaminoff, L. & Matthews, A. (2012) *Yoga Anatomy.* The Breathe Trust.

Lasater, J. H. (2009) *Yogabody: Anatomy, Kinesiology, and Asana.* Rodmell Press.

Long, R. (2010) *Anatomy for Arm Balances and Inversions.* Greenleaf Book Group.

Long, R. (2010) *Anatomy for Hip Openers and Forward Bends.* Bandha Yoga Publications.

Long, R. (2010) *Anatomy for Vinyasa Flow and Standing Poses.* Bandha Yoga Publications.

Long, R. (2008) *The Key Muscles of Yoga.* Raymond A. Long.

Peal, A. (n.d.) *Anatomy for Yogis.* www.yogaanytime.com/show-season/81/Yoga-Anatomy-for-Yogis-Season-1-Arturo-Peal.

AYURVEDA

Arora, l. (2022) *Soma: 100 Heritage Recipes for Self-Care.* YogSadhana.

Frawley, D. & Kozak, S. S. (2001) *Yoga for Your Type: An Ayurvedic Approach to Your Asana Practice.* Lotus.

Lad, V. (2012) *Textbook for Ayurveda: General Principles of Management and Treatment*, Vol. 3. The Ayurvedic Press.

Lad, V. (2007) *Textbook for Ayurveda: A Complete Guide to Clinical Assessment*, Vol. 2. The Ayurvedic Press.

Lad, V. (2002) *Textbook for Ayurveda: Fundamental Principles*, Vol. 1. The Ayurvedic Press.

Morrison, J. H. (2013) *The Book of Ayurveda: A Holistic Approach to Health and Longevity.* Touchstone.

Pole, S. (2013) *Ayurvedic Medicine: The Principles of Traditional Practice.* Singing Dragon.

Svoboda, R. E. (2011) *Prakriti: Your Ayurvedic Constitution.* Lotus Press.

CULTURAL APPROPRIATION

Jackson, L. M. (2019) *White Negroes: When Cornrows were in Vogue...and Other Thoughts on Cultural Appropriation.* Beacon Press.

HEALTH DISPARITIES

Beard, H. & Hoytt, E. H. (2012) *Health First! The Black Woman's Wellness Guide.* SmileyBooks.

Cooper, L. (2021) *Why Are Health Disparities Everyone's Problem?* Johns Hopkins University Press.

deShazo, R. D. (Ed.) (2018) *The Racial Divide in American Medicine: Black Physicians and the Struggle for Justice in Health Care.* [Electronic resource]. University Press of Mississippi.

O'Conner, B. (1994) *Healing Traditions: Alternative Medicine and the Health Professions (Studies in Health, Illness and Caregiving).* University of Pennsylvania Press.

Williams, M. T., Rosen, D. C., & Kanter, J. W. (Eds.) (2019) *Eliminating Race-Based Mental Health Disparities: Promoting Equity and Culturally Responsive Care Across Settings.* New Harbinger.

MEDITATION

Berila, B., Klein, M., & Roberts, C. J. (Eds.) (2016) *Yoga, The Body, and Embodied Social Change: An Intersectional Feminist Analysis.* Lexington Books.

Gates, R. & Kenison, K. (2002) *Meditations from the Mat: Daily Reflections on the Path of Yoga.* Anchor Books/Random House.

Gendlin, E. T. (1981) *Focusing.* Bantam Books.

Gunaratana, B. (2011) *Mindfulness in Plain English.* Wisdom Publications.

Hanh, T. N. (2019) *The Miracle of Mindfulness: An Introduction to the Practice of Meditation.* Beacon Press.

Harrell, S. The Soulfulness Center. www.thesoulfulnesscenter.com.

Harrell, S. (2022) Some loving kindness for your soul. www.thesoulfulnesscenter.com/post/some-loving-kindness-for-your-soul.

Harrell, S. P. (2018) Soulfulness as an orientation to contemplative practice: Culture, liberation, and mindful awareness. *Journal of Contemplative Inquiry* 5(1). https://digscholarship.unco.edu/joci/vol5/iss1/6.

Harrell, S. (n.d.) What is soulfulness. www.thesoulfulnesscenter.com/post/what-is-soulfulness.

Khalsa, D.S.Y. & Stauth, C. (2001) *Meditation as Medicine: Activate the Power of Your Natural Healing Force.* Fireside.

Singer, M. A. (2007) *The Untethered Soul: The Journey Beyond Yourself.* New Harbinger.

PERSONAL PRACTICE

Arora, l. (2022) *Soma: 100 Heritage Recipes for Self-Care.* YogSadhana.

Desai, K. (2010) *Life Lessons Love Lessons: A Guru's Daughter Discovers Knowledge is Only Half the Journey.* Red Elixir.

Desikachar, T. (1999) *The Heart of Yoga: Developing a Personal Practice.* Inner Traditions International.

Hafiz, S. (2018) *The Healing: One Woman's Journey from Poverty to Inner Riches.* Parallax Press.

Johnson, M. C. (2023) *We Heal Together: Rituals and Practices for Building Community and Connection.* Shambhala.

Lasater, J. H. (2015) *Living Your Yoga: Finding the Spiritual in Everyday Life.* Shambhala.

Smith, D. (2014) *Yes, Yoga Has Curves*, Vols. 1 & 2. Dana Smith.

PRANAYAMA

Brown, R. P. & Gerbarg, P. L. (2012) *The Healing Power of the Breath: Simple Techniques to Reduce Stress and Anxiety, Enhance Concentration, and Balance Your Emotions.* Shambhala.

Farhi, D. (1996) *The Breathing Book: Good Health and Vitality through Essential Breath Work.* Henry Holt and Company.

Iyengar, B.K.S. (2006) *Light on Pranayama: The Yogic Art of Breathing.* Crossroad Publishing Company.

Rosen, R. (2006) *Pranayama beyond the Fundamentals.* Shambhala.

Rosen, R. (2002) *The Yoga of Breath: A Step-by-Step Guide to Pranayama.* Shambhala.

RACE-BASED TRAUMA

Andersen, M. L. & Collins, P. H. (2019) *Race, Class & Gender: Intersections and Inequalities.* Cengage Learning.

Drake, St. C. & Cayton, H. R. (1945/2015) *Black Metropolis: A Study of Negro Life in a Northern City.* University of Chicago Press.

Jeffers-Coley, P. (2022) *We Got Soul, We Can Heal: Overcoming Racial Trauma through Leadership, Community and Resilience.* Toplight Books.

King, R. (2018) *Mindful of Race: Transforming Racism from the Inside Out.* Sounds True.

Menakem, R. (2017) *My Grandmother's Hands: Racialized Trauma and the Pathway to Mending Our Hearts and Bodies.* Central Recovery Press.

Myrdal, G. (1995) *An American Dilemma: The Negro Problem and Modern Democracy.* Routledge.

Parker, G. (2022) *Transforming Ethnic and Race-Based Traumatic Stress with Yoga.* Singing Dragon.

Parker, G. (2020) *Restorative Yoga for Ethnic and Race-Based Stress and Trauma.* Singing Dragon.

Wilkerson, I. (2020) *Caste: The Origins of Our Discontent.* Random House.

RESTORATIVE

Hersey, T. (2022) *Rest is Resistance: A Manifesto.* Little Brown Spark.

Lasater, J. H. (1995) *Relax and Renew: Restful Yoga for Stressful Times.* Rodmell Press.

Parker, G. (2022) *Transforming Ethnic and Race-Based Traumatic Stress with Yoga.* Singing Dragon.

Parker, G. (2020) *Restorative Yoga for Ethnic and Race-Based Stress and Trauma.* Singing Dragon.

Raheem, O. (2022) *Pause, Rest, Be: Stillness Practices for Courage in Times of Change.* Shambhala.

SPIRITUALITY

Boon, B. (2007) *Holy Yoga: Exercise for the Christian Body and Soul.* Holy Yoga Living.

Williams, A. K., Owens, L. R., & Syedullah, J. (2016) *Radical Dharma: Talking Race, Love, and Liberation.* North Atlantic Books.

Yetunde, P. A. (2020) *Black and Buddhist: What Buddhism Can Teach Us about Race, Resilience, Transformation, and Freedom.* Shambhala.

Zach, J., Smothers, D., & Chalfant, C. (2007) *Christian Yoga: Restoration for Body and Soul.* Hudson House.

TEACHING YOGA

Arora, I. (2019) *Yoga.* YogSadhana.

Bachman, N. (2004) *The Language of Yoga: Complete A to Y Guide to Asana Names, Sanskrit Terms, and Chants.* Sounds True.

Clark, B. (2012) *The Complete Guide to Yin Yoga.* White Cloud Press.

Dale, C. (2009) *The Subtle Body: An Encyclopedia of Your Energetic Anatomy.* Sounds True.

Fahri, D. (2006) *Teaching Yoga: Exploring the Teacher–Student Relationship.* Rodmell Press.

Grilley, P. (2012) *Yin Yoga: Principles and Practice.* White Cloud Press.

Ippoliti, A. & Smith, T. (2016) *The Art and Business of Teaching Yoga.* New World Library.

Khalsa, S.B.S., Cohen, L., McCall, T., & Telles, S. (Eds.) (2016) *The Principles and Practice of Yoga in Health Care.* Handspring Publishing.

Klein, M. C. (2018) *Yoga Rising: 30 Empowering Stories from Yoga Renegades for Every Body.* Llewellyn Publications.

Lasater, J. H. (2020) *Yoga Myths: What You Need to Learn and Unlearn for a Safe and Healthy Yoga Practice.* Shambhala Press.

LePage, J. & Aboim, L. (2020) *Yoga Toolbox Project for Teachers and Students.* Integrative Yoga. https://iytyogatherapy.com/product/1-toolbox.

McCall, T. (2007) *Yoga as Medicine: The Yogic Prescription for Health and Healing.* Bantam Books.

Stephens, M. (2014) *Yoga Adjustments: Philosophy, Principles, and Techniques.* North Atlantic Books.

Stephens, M. (2012) *Yoga Sequencing: Designing Transformative Yoga Classes.* North Atlantic Books.

Stephens, M. (2010) *Teaching Yoga: Essential Foundations and Techniques.* North Atlantic Books.

Weintraub, A. (2012) *Yoga Skills for Therapists: Effective Practices for Mood Management.* W. W. Norton.

YOGA NIDRA

Desai, K. (2017) *Yoga Nidra: The Art of Transformational Sleep.* First Lotus Press.

Miller, R. (2022) *Yoga Nidra: The iRest Meditative Practice for Deep Relaxation and Healing.* Sounds True.

Miller, R. (2015) *The iRest Program for Healing PTSD: A Proven Effective Approach to Using Yoga Nidra Meditation and Deep Relaxation Techniques to Overcome Trauma.* Harbinger Publications.

Satyananda, S. (2015) *Yoga Nidra.* Yoga Publications Trust.

Stanley, T. (2021) *Radiant Rest: Yoga Nidra for Deep Relaxation and Awakened Clarity.* Shambhala.

Tuli, U. D. (2014) *Yoni Shakti: A Woman's Guide to Power and Freedom through Yoga and Tantra.* YogaWords.

YOGA PHILOSOPHY

Adele, D. (2023) *The Kleshas: Exploring the Elusiveness of Happiness.* On-Word Bound Books.

Adele, D. (2009) *The Yamas & Niyamas: Exploring Yoga's Ethical Practice.* On-Word Bound Books.

DeLuca, E. (Ed.) (2003) *Pathways to Joy: The Master Vivekananda on the Four Yoga Paths to God.* Inner Ocean Publishing.

Easwaran, K. (2007) *The Dhammapada.* Nilgiri Press.

Easwaran, K. (2007) *The Upanishads.* 2nd Ed. Nilgiri Press.

Easwaran, K. (2000) *The Bhagavad Gita.* Nilgiri Press.

Judith, A. (2004) *Eastern Body Western Mind: Psychology and the Chakra System as a Path to the Self*. Random House.

Feurerstein, G. (2008) *The Yoga Tradition: Its History, Literature, Philosophy and Practice*. Hohm Press.

Iyengar, B.K.S. (2005) *Light on Life, the Yoga Journey to Wholeness, Inner Peace and Ultimate Freedom*. Rodale Press.

Little, T. (2020) *The Practice is the Path: Lessons and Reflections on the Transformative Power of Yoga*. Shambala.

Mewada, A., Keswani, J., Sharma, H., Tewani, G. R., & Nair, P.M.K. (2022) Ashtanga yoga ethics-based yoga versus general yoga on anthropometric indices, trigunas, and quality of life in abdominal obesity: a randomized control trial. *International Journal of Yoga* 15(2): 130–6.

Ranganthan, S. (2009) *Patanjali's Yoga Sutra*. Penguin Classics.

Satchidananda, S. S. (2007) *The Yoga Sutras of Patanjali*. Integral Yoga.

Whitwell, M. (2004) *Yoga of Heart: The Healing Power of Intimate Connection*. Lantern Books.

Yogapedia. (n.d) Mudra. www.yogapedia.com/the-best-of-the-mudras/2/7371.

Endnotes

INTRODUCTION

1   Schrein, C. M. (2015) Lucy: A marvelous specimen. *Nature Education Knowledge* 6(7): 2.

2   Carrera, J. (2006) *Inside the Yoga Sutras: A Comprehensive Sourcebook for the Study and Practice of Patanjali's Yoga Sutras.* Integral Yoga Publications, p. 4.

3   Chissell, J. T. (2000) *Pyramids of Power! An Ancient African Centered Approach to Optimal Health.* Positive Perceptions Publications, p. 4.

4   Carrera, J. (2006) *Inside the Yoga Sutras: A Comprehensive Sourcebook for the Study and Practice of Patanjali's Yoga Sutras.* Integral Yoga Publications, p. 152.

5   Centers for Disease Control and Prevention (1997) *CDC-Kaiser Permanente Adverse Childhood Experiences (ACE Study).* www.cdc.gov/violenceprevention/aces/about. html.

6   Menakem, R. (2017) *My Grandmother's Hands: Racialized Trauma and the Pathway to Mending Our Hearts and Bodies.* Central Recovery Press, p. 28.

7   Lee, M. (2014) *Working the Roots: Over 400 Years of Traditional African American Healing.* Wadastick Publishers, p. ix.

CHAPTER 1

1   Morris, W. (Ed.) (1982) *The American Heritage Dictionary of the English Language: New College Edition.* Houghton Mifflin Company, p. 607.

2   Morris, W. (Ed.) (1982) *The American Heritage Dictionary of the English Language: New College Edition.* Houghton Mifflin Company, p. 607.

3   Egnew, T. R. (2005) The meaning of healing: transcending suffering. *Annals of Family Medicine* 3(3): 255.

4   Morris, W. (Ed.) (1982) *The American Heritage Dictionary of the English Language: New College Edition.* Houghton Mifflin Company, p. 1520.

5   Carrera, J. (2006) *Inside the Yoga Sutras: A Comprehensive Sourcebook for the Study and Practice of Patanjali's Yoga Sutras.* Integral Yoga Publications, p. 368.

6   Mobe, T. (2002) 8 African proverbs every global citizen should know. *Global Citizen.* www.globalcitizen.org/en/content/africa-proverbs-global-citizens-action-end-poverty.

7   Thich, N. H. (2002) What is Sangha? *Lion's Roar.* www.lionsroar.com/the-practice-of-sangha.

8   Elliott, M. & Hughes, J. (2019, August 19) Four hundred years after enslaved Africans were first brought to Virginia, most Americans still don't know the full story of slavery. *New York Times Magazine's 1619 Project.* www.nytimes.com/interactive/2019/08/19/magazine/history-slavery-smithsonian.html.

9   Mitchem, S. Y. (2017) *African American Folk Healing*. New York University Press, p. 15.

10 Carrera, J. (2006) *Inside the Yoga Sutras: A Comprehensive Sourcebook for the Study and Practice of Patanjali's Yoga Sutras*. Integral Yoga Publications, p. 205.

CHAPTER 2

1   Allard, S. (2021, July 15) What is kirtan? *Hinduamerican*. www.hinduamerican.org/blog/what-is-kirtan.

2   Mitchem, S. Y. (2017) *African American Folk Healing*. New York University Press, p. 20.

3   Mamiya, L. (1999) The Black Church. In Appiah, K. A. & Gates, Jr., H. L. (Eds.) *Africana: The Encyclopedia of the African and African American Experience*. Basic Civitas Books, pp. 241–5.

4   Mokgobi, M. G. (2014) Understanding traditional African healing. *African Journal for Physical Health Education, Recreation and Dance* 20(Suppl. 2): 24–34.

5   Cotton, S., Luberto, C. M., Yi, M. S., & Tsevat, J. (2011) Complementary and alternative medicine behaviors and beliefs in urban adolescents with asthma. *Journal of Asthma* 48(5): 531–8. https://pubmed.ncbi.nlm.nih.gov/21504264.

6   Shani, P. & Walter, E. (2022) Acceptability and use of mind-body interventions among African American cancer survivors: an integrative review. *Integrative Cancer Therapy*. https://pubmed.ncbi.nlm.nih.gov/35786041.

7   National Center for Complimentary and Integrative Health (n.d.) *Herbs at a Glance*. www.nccih.nih.gov/health/herbsataglance.

8   Covey, H. C. (2007) *African American Slave Medicine: Herbal and Non-Herbal Treatments*. Lexington Books, pp. 162, 175.

9   Covey, H. C. (2007) *African American Slave Medicine: Herbal and Non-Herbal Treatments*. Lexington Books, p. 162.

10 Frawley, D. & Lad, V. (2001) *The Yoga of Herbs: An Ayurvedic Guide to Herbal Medicine*. 2nd Ed. Lotus Press, p. xi.

11 Mills, S. Y. (1991) *The Essential Book of Herbal Medicine*. Penguin Press, p. 194.

12 Barnett, M. C., Cotroneo, M., Purnell, J., Martin, D., *et al.* (2003) Use of CAM in local African American communities: community-partnered research. *Journal of the National Medical Association* 95(10): 943, 950.

13 We Are Wanda (n.d.) *Women Advancing Nutrition, Dietetics and Agriculture*. www.iamwanda.org.

14 Porges, S. (2021, June 17–19) Ancient wisdom meets contemporary neuroscience: yoga through the lens of polyvagal theory. Symposium on yoga therapy and research, International Association of Yoga Therapists.

15 Sayeed, S. A. & Prakash, A. (2013) The Islamic prayer (Salah/Namaaz) and yoga togetherness in mental health. *Indian Journal of Psychiatry* 55(Suppl. 2): S224–S230.

16 Hwang, P. W. & Braun, K. L. (2015) The effectiveness of dance interventions to improve older adults' health: a systematic literature review. *Alternative Therapies in Health and Medicine* 21(5): 64–70.

17 Lacy, M. D. & Zucker, A. (2006, August 28) *Free to Dance*. Great Performances: Dance in America. www.thirteen.org/freetodance/about/index.html#:~:text=Great%20Performance.

18 Dunham, K. (1969) *Island Possessed*. University of Chicago Press, p. 109.

19 Tyrus, J. & Novosel, P. (2021) *Dance Theatre of Harlem: A History, a Movement, a Celebration*. Kensington Publishing Corporation, p. 86.

20 Wignot, J. (Director) & DeFillipe, L. (Producer) (2021) *Ailey*. Documentary. Insignia Films. https://insigniafilms.com/Ailey.

21 Zollar, J.W.J. (2018) *Urban Bush Women*. www.urbanbushwomen.org.

22 Ozuzu, O. (Host) (2013, October 24) *Bill T. Jones: A Life Well Danced.* Chicago Humanities Festival. www.youtube.com/watch?v=QfvUYqJjQbs.

23 Hurston, Z. N. (1938) *Tell My Horse: Voodoo and Life in Haiti and Jamaica.* Amistad Press, p. 113.

24 Le Peristyle Haitian Sanctuary (n.d) Home page. www.lpshpa.com.

25 Le Peristyle Haitian Sanctuary (n.d) Home page. www.lpshpa.com.

26 Harvard Divinity School (2021, December 14) *Black Magic Matters: Hoodoo as Ancestral Religion: A Conversation with Yvonne Chireau.* Video. Center for the Study of World Religions. https://cswr.hds.harvard.edu/news/magic-matters/2021/11/10.

27 Alvarado, D. (n.d.) Home page. Crossroads University. www.crossroadsuniversity.com.

28 Anderson, J. E. (2005) *Conjure in African American Society.* Louisiana State University Press, p. 49.

CHAPTER 3

1   Lee, M. E. (2017) *Working the Root: Over 400 Years of Traditional African American Healing.* Wadastick Publishers, p. xiii.

2   Mitchem, S. Y. (2017) *African American Folk Healing.* New York University Press, p. 29.

3   Muhammad, E. (1967) *How to Eat to Live, Book One.* Final Call Press, p. 22.

4   Muhammad, E. (1967) *How to Eat to Live, Book One.* Final Call Press, p. 57.

5   Gregory, D. (1973) *Dick Gregory's Natural Diet for Folks Who Eat: Cookin' with Mother Nature.* Harper & Row Publishers, p. 89.

6   Afrika, L. O. (1983) *African Holistic Health.* Adesegun, Johnson and Koram Publishers, p. 2.

7   Edwards, C. (2019, June 8) *Dr Sebi Documentary.* www.youtube.com/watch?v=9ycV9aAWjzM.

8   Gullah Geechee Herbal Gathering (n.d.) Home page. www.gullahgeecheeherbs.org.

9   Berkman, F. J. (2010) *Monument Eternal: The Music of Alice Coltrane.* Wesleyan University Press, p. 9.

10 Carrera, J. (2006) *Inside the Yoga Sutras: A Comprehensive Sourcebook for the Study and Practice of Patanjali's Yoga Sutras.* Integral Yoga Publications, p. 98.

11 3HO. *About Kundalini Yoga.* www.3ho.org/more-about-kundalini-yoga.

12 Kaur, K. (n.d.) About Krishna Kaur. www.krishnakaur.org/about.

13 Hotep, Y. R. (n.d.) *What is Kemetic Yoga?* https://kemeticyogaskills.com/what-is-kemetic-yoga.

14 Ashby, S. M. (2005) *Egyptian Yoga: The Philosophy of Enlightenment*, Vol. 1. 10th anniversary Ed. Cruzian Mystic Books, p. 66.

15 Ashby, S. M. (2005) *Egyptian Yoga: The Philosophy of Enlightenment*, Vol. 1. 10th anniversary Ed. Cruzian Mystic Books, p. 66.

16 Eddie, F. (producer) (2021, March 23) *Queen Afua & SupaNova Slom on Ultimate Healing of the Mind, Body & Spirit, Feminine Wellness + More.* Breakfast Club Podcast. www.youtube.com/watch?v=kGVtye47wqo.

17 Black Yoga Teachers Alliance (n.d.) Home page. https://blackyogateachersalliance.org/who-we-are.

18 Chissell, J. T. (2000) *Pyramids of Power! An Ancient African Centered Approach to Optimal Health.* Positive Perceptions Publications, p. xiv.

19 Evans, M. C., Bazargan, M., Cobb, S., & Assari, S. (2019) Pain intensity among community-dwelling African American older adults in an economically disadvantaged area of Los Angeles: social, behavioral, and health determinants. *International Journal of Environmental Research and Public Health* 16: 3894.

20 Orhan, C., Looveren, E. V., Cagnie, B., Mukhtar, N. B., *et al.* (2018) Are pain beliefs, cognitions, and behaviors influenced by race, ethnicity, and culture in patients with chronic musculoskeletal pain: a systematic review. *Pain Physician Journal* 21: 541–58.

21 Mills, S. & Boone, K. (2000) *Principles and Practice of Phytotherapy: Modern Herbal Medicine.* Churchill Livingstone, p. 22.

22 Barnett, M. C., Cotroneo, M., Purnell, J., Martin, D., *et al.* (2003) Use of CAM in local African American communities: community-partnered research. *Journal of the National Medical Association* 95(10): 943–50.

23 Middleton, K. R., Ward, M. M., Moonaz, S. H., Lopez, M. M., *et al.* (2018) Feasibility and assessment of outcome measures for yoga as self-care for minorities with arthritis: a pilot study. *Pilot & Feasibility Studies* 4: 53.

24 Chissell, J. T. (2000) *Pyramids of Power! An Ancient African Centered Approach to Optimal Health.* Positive Perceptions Publications, p. xiv.

PART II

1   Gaston, G. B. (2013) African-Americans' perceptions of health care provider cultural competence that promote HIV medical self-care and antiretroviral medication adherence. *AIDS Care* 25(9): 1159–65.

CHAPTER 4

1   Centers for Disease Control and Prevention (2022) *Advancing Health Equity in Chronic Disease Prevention and Management.* www.cdc.gov/chronicdisease/healthequity/index.htm.

2   Kullar, R., Marcelin, J. R., Swartz, T. H., Piggott, D. A., *et al.* (2020) Racial disparity of coronavirus disease 2019 in African American communities. *The Journal of Infectious Diseases* 222(6): 890–3.

3   American Public Health Association (2022) *Racism and Health 2022.* www.apha.org/topics-and-issues/health-equity/racism-and-health.

4   American Public Health Association (2022) *Racism and Health, 2022.* www.apha.org/topics-and-issues/health-equity/racism-and-health.

5   Banaji, M. R., Fiske, S. T., & Massey, D. S. (2021) Systemic racism: individual and interactions, institutions and society. *Cognitive Research: Principles and Implications* 6: art. 82, p. 1.

6   Banaji, M. R., Fiske, S. T., & Massey, D. S. (2021) Systemic racism: individual and interactions, institutions and society. *Cognitive Research: Principles and Implications* 6: art. 82, p. 1.

7   Hill-Briggs, F., Ephraim, P. L., Vrany, E. A., Davidson, K. W., *et al.* (2022) Social determinates of health, race, and diabetes population health improvement: Black/African Americans as a population exemplar. *Current Diabetes Reports* 22: 117–25, p. 120.

8   Lim, D. (2020, May 10) I'm embracing the term "people of global majority." *Medium.* https://regenerative.medium.com/im-embracing-the-term-people-of-the-global-majority-abd1c1251241.

9   Department of Health and Human Services (2022) *HHS Equity Action Plan.* www.hhs.gov/sites/default/files/hhs-equity-action-plan.pdf.

10 Beech, B. M., Ford, C., Thorpe, R. J. Jr., Bruce, M. A., & Norris, K. C. (2021) Poverty, racism, and the public health crisis in America. *Frontiers of Public Health* 9: 699049, p. 2.

11 Beech, B. M., Ford, C., Thorpe, R. J. Jr., Bruce, M. A., & Norris, K. C. (2021) Poverty, racism, and the public health crisis in America. *Frontiers of Public Health* 9: 699049, pp. 2–3.

12 Hoffman, K. M., Trawalter, S., Axt, J. R., & Oliver, M. N. (2016) Racial bias in pain assessment and treatment recommendations, and false beliefs about biological differences between blacks and whites. *Proceedings of the National Academy of Sciences of the United States of America* 113(16): 4296–301.

13 Beech, B. M., Ford, C., Thorpe, R. J. Jr., Bruce, M. A., & Norris, K. C. (2021) Poverty, racism, and the public health crisis in America. *Frontiers of Public Health* 9: 699049, pp. 2–3.

14 Beech, B. M., Ford, C., Thorpe, R. J. Jr., Bruce, M. A., & Norris, K. C. (2021) Poverty, racism, and the public health crisis in America. *Frontiers of Public Health* 9: 699049, pp. 2–3.

15 Beech, B. M., Ford, C., Thorpe, R. J. Jr., Bruce, M. A., & Norris, K. C. (2021) Poverty, racism, and the public health crisis in America. *Frontiers of Public Health* 9: 699049, p. 3.

16 Beech, B. M., Ford, C., Thorpe, R. J. Jr., Bruce, M. A., & Norris, K. C. (2021) Poverty, racism, and the public health crisis in America. *Frontiers of Public Health* 9: 699049, p. 3.

17 Beech, B. M., Ford, C., Thorpe, R. J. Jr., Bruce, M. A., & Norris, K. C. (2021) Poverty, racism, and the public health crisis in America. *Frontiers of Public Health* 9: 699049, p. 3.

CHAPTER 5

1 Department of Health and Human Services (2022) *HHS Equity Action Plan.* www.hhs.gov/sites/default/files/hhs-equity-action-plan.pdf.

2 Semega, J., Kollar, M., Creamer, J., & Mohanty, A. (2019) *Income and Poverty in the United States: 2019–Current Population Reports.* United States Census Bureau. www.census.gov/library/visualizations/2020/demo/p60-270.html.

3 Fashaw-Walters, S. (2022) *"Out of Reach": Inequities in Access to High-Quality Home Health Agencies.* Health Affairs Symposium on Racism and Health. www.healthaffairs.org/racism-and-health.

4 Homan, P. & Brown, T. (2022) Sick and Tired of being excluded: Structural racism in disenfranchisement as a threat to population health equity. *Health Affairs* 41(2). www.healthaffairs.org/doi/10.1377/hlthaff.2021.01414

5 Department of Health and Human Services (2022) *HHS Equity Action Plan.* www.hhs.gov/sites/default/files/hhs-equity-action-plan.pdf.

CHAPTER 6

1 Mendez, D. D., Scott, J., Adodoadji, L., Toval, C., McNeil, M., & Sindhu, J. (2021) Racism as public health crisis: assessment and review of municipal declarations and resolutions across the United States. *Frontiers in Public Health* 9: 686807.

2 Mendez, D. D., Scott, J., Adodoadji, L., Toval, C., McNeil, M., & Sindhu, J. (2021) Racism as public health crisis: assessment and review of municipal declarations and resolutions across the United States. *Frontiers in Public Health* 9: 686807.

3 George, M., Bruzzese, J.-M., Sommers, M. S., Pantalon, M. V., *et al.* (2021) Group-randomized trial of tailored brief shared decision-making to improve asthma control in urban black adults. *Journal of Advanced Nursing* 77(3): 1501–17, p. 3.

4 Santino, T. A., Chaves, G.S.S., Freitas, D. A., Fregonezi, G.A.F., & Mendonça, K.M.P.P. (2020) Breathing exercises for adults with asthma. *Cochrane Database of Systematic Reviews, Issue 3*: art. CD001277.

5   Hughes, H. K., Matsui, E. C., Tschudy, M. M., Pollack, C. E., & Keet, C. A. (2017) Pediatric asthma health disparities: race, hardship, housing, and asthma in a national survey. *Academic Pediatrics* 17(2): 127–34.

6   George, M., Bruzzese, J.-M., Sommers, M. S., Pantalon, M. V., *et al.* (2021) Group-randomized trial of tailored brief shared decision-making to improve asthma control in urban black adults. *Journal of Advanced Nursing* 77(3): 1501–17, p. 3.

7   Sangeethalaxmi, M. J. & Hankey, A. (2022) Impact of yoga breathing and relaxation as an add-on therapy on quality of life, anxiety, depression and pulmonary function in your adults with bronchial asthma: a randomized controlled trial. *Journal of Ayurveda and Integrative Medicine* 14: art. 100546.

8   Santino, T. A., Chaves, G.S.S., Freitas, D. A., Fregonezi, G.A.F., & Mendonça, K.M.P.P. (2020) Breathing exercises for adults with asthma. *Cochrane Database of Systematic Reviews, Issue 3*: art. CD001277.

9   Brown, R. P. & Gerbarg, P. L. (2012) *The Healing Power of the Breath: Simple Techniques to Reduce Stress and Anxiety, Enhance Concentration, and Balance Your Emotions*. Shambhala.

10 Jayawardena, R., Ranasinghe, P., Ranawaka, H., Gamage, N., Dissanayake, D., & Misra, A. (2020) Exploring the therapeutic benefits of pranayama (yogic breathing): a systematic review. *International Journal of Yoga* 13(2): 99–110.

11 Khalsa, S.B.S., Cohen, L., McCall, T., & Telles, S. (2016) *The Principles and Practice of Yoga in Health Care*. Handspring Publishing, p. 319.

12 Stoodley, I., Williams, L., Thompson, C., Scott, H., & Wood, L. (2019) Evidence for lifestyle interventions in asthma. *Breathe* 15: e50–e61

13 Barnes L. L. (2022) Alzheimer disease in African American individuals: increased incidence or not enough data? *Nature Reviews: Neurology* 18(1): 56–62.

14 Shaw, A. R., Perales-Puchalt, J., Moore, T., Weatherspoon, P., *et al.* (2022) Recruitment of older African Americans in Alzheimer's disease clinical trials using a community education approach. *The Journal of Prevention of Alzheimer's Disease* 9(4): 672–8.

15 Shaw, A. R., Perales-Puchalt, J., Moore, T., Weatherspoon, P., *et al.* (2022) Recruitment of older African Americans in Alzheimer's disease clinical trials using a community education approach. *The Journal of Prevention of Alzheimer's Disease* 9(4): 672–8.

16 Alzheimer's Research and Prevention Foundation (n.d.) Home page. https://alzheimersprevention.org.

17 Lavretsky, H., Epel, W. S., Siddarth, P., Nazarian, N., *et al.* (2013) A pilot study of yogic meditation for family dementia caregivers with depressive symptoms: effects on mental health, cognition, and telomerase activity. *International Journal of Geriatric Psychiatry* 28: 57–65.

18 Chinn, J. J., Martin, I. K., & Redmond, N. (2021) Health equity among black women in the United States. *Journal of Women's Health* 30(2): 212–19.

19 Spinner, J. R. (2022) An examination of the impact of social and cultural traditions contributing to overweight and obesity among black women. *Journal of Primary Care & Community Health* 13: 1–8, p. 6.

20 Stoodley, I., Williams, L., Thompson, C., Scott, H., & Wood, L. (2019) Evidence for lifestyle interventions in asthma. *Breathe* 15: e50–e61.

21 Spinner, J. R. (2022) An examination of the impact of social and cultural traditions contributing to overweight and obesity among black women. *Journal of Primary Care & Community Health* 13: 1–8, p. 1.

22 Spinner, J. R. (2022) An examination of the impact of social and cultural traditions contributing to overweight and obesity among black women. *Journal of Primary Care & Community Health* 13: 1–8, p. 1.

23 Spinner, J. R. (2022) An examination of the impact of social and cultural traditions contributing to overweight and obesity among black women. *Journal of Primary Care & Community Health* 13: 1–8, p. 1.

24 Spinner, J. R. (2022) An examination of the impact of social and cultural traditions contributing to overweight and obesity among black women. *Journal of Primary Care & Community Health* 13: 1–8, p. 2.

25 Spinner, J. R. (2022) An examination of the impact of social and cultural traditions contributing to overweight and obesity among black women. *Journal of Primary Care & Community Health* 13: 1–8, p. 6.

26 Spinner, J. R. (2022) An examination of the impact of social and cultural traditions contributing to overweight and obesity among black women. *Journal of Primary Care & Community Health* 13: 1–8, p. 1.

27 Weir, C. B. & Jan, A. (2022) BMI classification percentile and cut off points. In *StatPearls*. StatPearls Publishing.

28 Bray, G. A. (2023) Beyond BMI. *Nutrients* 15(10): 2254.

29 Spinner, J. R. (2022) An examination of the impact of social and cultural traditions contributing to overweight and obesity among black women. *Journal of Primary Care & Community Health* 13: 1–8, p. 1.

30 Spinner, J. R. (2022) An examination of the impact of social and cultural traditions contributing to overweight and obesity among black women. *Journal of Primary Care & Community Health* 13: 1–8, p. 2.

31 Spinner, J. R. (2022) An examination of the impact of social and cultural traditions contributing to overweight and obesity among black women. *Journal of Primary Care & Community Health* 13: 1–8, p. 6.

32 Rioux, J. & Howerter, A. (2019) Outcomes from a whole-systems Ayurvedic medicine and yoga therapy treatment for obesity pilot study. *Journal of Alternative and Complementary Medicine* 25(Suppl. 1): S124–S137.

33 Liu, Y., Qu, H. Q., Qu, J., Chang, X., *et al.* (2022) Burden of rare coding variants reveals genetic heterogeneity between obese and non-obese asthma patients in the African American population. *Respiratory Research* 23(1): 116

34 Khalsa, S.B.S., Cohen, L., McCall, T., & Telles, S. (2016) *The Principles and Practice of Yoga in Health Care.* Handspring Publishing, p. 319.

35 Webb, J. B., Padro, M. P., Thomas, E. V., Davies, A. E., *et al.* (2022) Yoga at every size: a preliminary evaluation of a brief online size-inclusive yoga and body gratitude journaling intervention to enhance positive embodiment in higher weight college women. *Frontiers in Global Womens Health* 3: art. 852854.

36 Lee, C., Park, S., & Boylan, J. J. (2020) Cardiovascular health at the intersection of race and gender: identifying life-course processes to reduce health disparities. *The Journals of Gerontology: Series B* 76(6): 1127–39.

37 Lee, C., Park, S., & Boylan, J. J. (2020) Cardiovascular health at the intersection of race and gender: identifying life-course processes to reduce health disparities. *The Journals of Gerontology: Series B* 76(6): 1127–39, p. 1127.

38 Lee, C., Park, S., & Boylan, J. J. (2020) Cardiovascular health at the intersection of race and gender: identifying life-course processes to reduce health disparities. *The Journals of Gerontology: Series B* 76(6): 1127–39.

39 Henry, T. L., Jetty, A., Petterson, S., Jaffree, H., *et al.* (2020) Taking a closer look at mental health treatment differences: effectiveness of mental health treatment by provider type in racial and ethnic minorities. *Journal of Primary Care & Community Health* 11.

40 Lee, C., Park, S., & Boylan, J. J. (2020) Cardiovascular health at the intersection of race and gender: identifying life-course processes to reduce health disparities. *The Journals of Gerontology: Series B* 76(6): 1127–39, p. 1129.

41 Khalsa, S.B.S., Cohen, L., McCall, T., & Telles, S. (2016) *The Principles and Practice of Yoga in Health Care.* Handspring Publishing, p. 319.

42 Guidi, J., Lucente, M., Sonino, N., & Fava, G. A. (2021) Allostatic load and its impact on health: a systematic review. *Psychotherapy and Psychosomatics* 90(1): 11–27.

43 Hill-Briggs, F., Ephraim, P. L., Vrany, E. A., Davidson, K. W., *et al.* (2022) Social determinates of health, race, and diabetes population health improvement: Black/ African Americans as a population exemplar. *Current Diabetes Reports* 22: 117–25, p. 119.

44 Ng, M.C.Y. (2015) Genetics of type 2 diabetes in African Americans. *Current Diabetes Reports* 15: 74.

45 Hill-Briggs, F., Ephraim, P. L., Vrany, E. A., Davidson, K. W., *et al.* (2022) Social determinates of health, race, and diabetes population health improvement: Black/ African Americans as a population exemplar. *Current Diabetes Reports* 22: 117–25, p. 118

46 Hill-Briggs, F., Ephraim, P. L., Vrany, E. A., Davidson, K. W., *et al.* (2022) Social determinates of health, race, and diabetes population health improvement: Black/ African Americans as a population exemplar. *Current Diabetes Reports* 22: 117–25, p. 119

47 Hill-Briggs, F., Ephraim, P. L., Vrany, E. A., Davidson, K. W., *et al.* (2022) Social determinates of health, race, and diabetes population health improvement: Black/ African Americans as a population exemplar. *Current Diabetes Reports* 22: 117–25, p. 119

48 Hill-Briggs, F., Ephraim, P. L., Vrany, E. A., Davidson, K. W., *et al.* (2022) Social determinates of health, race, and diabetes population health improvement: Black/ African Americans as a population exemplar. *Current Diabetes Reports* 22: 117–25, p. 120

49 Hill-Briggs, F., Ephraim, P. L., Vrany, E. A., Davidson, K. W., *et al.* (2022) Social determinates of health, race, and diabetes population health improvement: Black/ African Americans as a population exemplar. *Current Diabetes Reports* 22: 117–25, p. 120

50 Hill-Briggs, F., Ephraim, P. L., Vrany, E. A., Davidson, K. W., *et al.* (2022) Social determinates of health, race, and diabetes population health improvement: Black/ African Americans as a population exemplar. *Current Diabetes Reports* 22: 117–25, p. 120

51 Ng, M.C.Y. (2015) Genetics of type 2 diabetes in African Americans. *Current Diabetes Reports* 15: 74.

52 Khalsa, S.B.S., Cohen, L., McCall, T., & Telles, S. (2016) *The Principles and Practice of Yoga in Health Care.* Handspring Publishing, p. 319.

53 Abel, W. E. & DeHaven, H. J. (2021) An interactive technology enhanced coaching intervention for Black women with hypertension: randomized controlled trial study protocol. *Research in Nursing and Health* 44(1), p. 10.

54 Abel, W. E. & DeHaven, H. J. (2021) An interactive technology enhanced coaching intervention for Black women with hypertension: randomized controlled trial study protocol. *Research in Nursing and Health* 44(1), p. 2.

55 Abel, W. E. & DeHaven, H. J. (2021) An interactive technology enhanced coaching intervention for Black women with hypertension: randomized controlled trial study protocol. *Research in Nursing and Health* 44(1), p. 1.

56 Abel, W. E. & DeHaven, H. J. (2021) An interactive technology enhanced coaching intervention for Black women with hypertension: randomized controlled trial study protocol. *Research in Nursing and Health* 44(1), p. 11.

57 Abel, W. E. & DeHaven, H. J. (2021) An interactive technology enhanced coaching intervention for Black women with hypertension: randomized controlled trial study protocol. *Research in Nursing and Health* 44(1), p. 2.

58 Khalsa, S.B.S., Cohen, L., McCall, T., & Telles, S. (2016) *The Principles and Practice of Yoga in Health Care.* Handspring Publishing, p. 300.

59 Hill-Briggs, F., Ephraim, P. L., Vrany, E. A., Davidson, K. W., *et al.* (2022) Social determinates of health, race, and diabetes population health improvement: Black/African Americans as a population exemplar. *Current Diabetes Reports* 22: 117–25, p. 120.

60 Williams, D. R. (2018) Stress and the mental health of populations of color: advancing our understanding of race-related stressors. *Journal of Health and Social Behavior* 59(4): 466–85, p. 2.

61 Henry, T. L., Jetty, A., Petterson, S., Jaffree, H., *et al.* (2020) Taking a closer look at mental health treatment differences: effectiveness of mental health treatment by provider type in racial and ethnic minorities. *Journal of Primary Care & Community Health* 11.

62 Han, E., & Liu, G. G. (2005) Racial disparities in prescription drug use for mental illness among population in US. *The Journal of Mental Health Policy and Economics* 8(3): 131–43.

63 American Psychological Association (n.d) "Mental Health." *APA Dictionary of Psychology.* https://dictionary.apa.org/mental-health.

64 Beech, B. M., Ford, C., Thorpe Jr., R. J. Bruce, M. A., & Norris, K. C. (2021) Poverty, racism, and the public health crisis in America. *Frontiers in Public Health* 9: art. 699049.

65 Chinn, J. J., Martin, I. K., & Redmond, N. (2021) Health equity among Black women in the United States. *Journal of Women's Health* 30(2): 212–19, p. 215.

66 Schmalzl, L., Powers, C., & Blom, E. H. (2015) Neurophysiological and neuro-cognitive mechanisms underlying the effects of yoga-based practices: towards a comprehensive theoretical framework. *Frontiers in Human Neuroscience* 9: art. 235.

67 Henry, T. L., Jetty, A., Petterson, S., Jaffree, H., *et al.* (2020) Taking a closer look at mental health treatment differences: effectiveness of mental health treatment by provider type in racial and ethnic minorities. *Journal of Primary Care & Community Health* 11.

68 Henry, T. L., Jetty, A., Petterson, S., Jaffree, H., *et al.* (2020) Taking a closer look at mental health treatment differences: effectiveness of mental health treatment by provider type in racial and ethnic minorities. *Journal of Primary Care & Community Health* 11.

69 Henry, T. L., Jetty, A., Petterson, S., Jaffree, H., *et al.* (2020) Taking a closer look at mental health treatment differences: effectiveness of mental health treatment by provider type in racial and ethnic minorities. *Journal of Primary Care & Community Health* 11.

70 Henry, T. L., Jetty, A., Petterson, S., Jaffree, H., *et al.* (2020) Taking a closer look at mental health treatment differences: effectiveness of mental health treatment by provider type in racial and ethnic minorities. *Journal of Primary Care & Community Health* 11.

71 Henry, T. L., Jetty, A., Petterson, S., Jaffree, H., *et al.* (2020) Taking a closer look at mental health treatment differences: effectiveness of mental health treatment by provider type in racial and ethnic minorities. *Journal of Primary Care & Community Health* 11.

72 Henry, T. L., Jetty, A., Petterson, S., Jaffree, H., *et al.* (2020) Taking a closer look at mental health treatment differences: effectiveness of mental health treatment by provider type in racial and ethnic minorities. *Journal of Primary Care & Community Health* 11.

73 Williams, D. R. (2018) Stress and the mental health of populations of color: advancing our understanding of race-related stressors. *Journal of Health and Social Behavior* 59(4): 466–85, p. 19.

74 Khalsa, S.B.S., Cohen, L., McCall, T., & Telles, S. (2016) *The Principles and Practice of Yoga in Health Care.* Handspring Publishing, p. 319.

75 Hoffman, K. M., Trawalter, S., Axt, J. R., & Oliver, M. N. (2016) Racial bias in pain assessment and treatment recommendations, and false beliefs about biological differences between blacks and whites. *Proceedings of the National Academy of Sciences of the United States of America* 113(16): 4296–301.

76 Green, C. R., Anderson, K. O., Baker, T. A., Campbell, L. C., *et al.* (2003) The unequal burden of pain: confronting racial and ethnic disparities in pain. *Pain Medicine* 4(3), p. 277.

77 Green, C. R., Anderson, K. O., Baker, T. A., Campbell, L. C., *et al.* (2003) The unequal burden of pain: confronting racial and ethnic disparities in pain. *Pain Medicine* 4(3), p. 278.

78 Green, C. R., Anderson, K. O., Baker, T. A., Campbell, L. C., *et al.* (2003) The unequal burden of pain: confronting racial and ethnic disparities in pain. *Pain Medicine* 4(3), p. 279.

79 Green, C. R., Anderson, K. O., Baker, T. A., Campbell, L. C., *et al.* (2003) The unequal burden of pain: confronting racial and ethnic disparities in pain. *Pain Medicine* 4(3), p. 280.

80 Khalsa, S.B.S., Cohen, L., McCall, T., & Telles, S. (2016) *The Principles and Practice of Yoga in Health Care.* Handspring Publishing.

81 Henry, T. L., Jetty, A., Petterson, S., Jaffree, H., *et al.* (2020) Taking a closer look at mental health treatment differences: effectiveness of mental health treatment by provider type in racial and ethnic minorities. *Journal of Primary Care & Community Health* 11, p. 1137.

82 Kullar, R., Marcelin, J. R., Swartz, T. H., Piggott, D. A., *et al.* (2020) Racial disparity of coronavirus disease 2019 in African American communities. *The Journal of Infectious Diseases* 22: 890–3, p. 890.

83 Kullar, R., Marcelin, J. R., Swartz, T. H., Piggott, D. A., *et al.* (2020) Racial disparity of coronavirus disease 2019 in African American communities. *The Journal of Infectious Diseases* 22: 890–3, p. 891.

84 Phillips, N., Park, I.-W., Robinson, J. R., & Jones, H. P. (2021) The perfect storm: COVID-19 health disparities in US blacks. *Journal of Racial and Ethnic Health Disparities* 8(5): 1153–60.

85 Phillips, N., Park, I.-W., Robinson, J. R., & Jones, H. P. (2021) The perfect storm: COVID-19 health disparities in US blacks. *Journal of Racial and Ethnic Health Disparities* 8(5): 1153–60.

86 Kullar, R., Marcelin, J. R., Swartz, T. H., Piggott, D. A., *et al.* (2020) Racial disparity of coronavirus disease 2019 in African American communities. *The Journal of Infectious Diseases* 22: 890–3, p. 891.

87 Poulson, M., Geary, A., Annesi, C., Allee, L., *et al.* (2021) National disparities in COVID-19 outcomes between black and white Americans. *Journal of the National Medical Association* 113(2): 125–32, p. 125.

88 Poulson, M., Geary, A., Annesi, C., Allee, L., *et al.* (2021) National disparities in COVID-19 outcomes between black and white Americans. *Journal of the National Medical Association* 113(2): 125–32, p. 131.

89 Phillips, N., Park, I.-W., Robinson, J. R., & Jones, H. P. (2021) The perfect storm: COVID-19 health disparities in US blacks. *Journal of Racial and Ethnic Health Disparities* 8(5): 1153–60.

90 Chinn, J. J., Martin, I. K., & Redmond, N. (2021) Health equity among black women in the United States. *Journal of Women's Health* 30(2): 212–19, p. 212.

91 Chinn, J. J., Martin, I. K., & Redmond, N. (2021) Health equity among black women in the United States. *Journal of Women's Health* 30(2): 212–19.

92 Chinn, J. J., Martin, I. K., & Redmond, N. (2021) Health equity among black women in the United States. *Journal of Women's Health* 30(2): 212–19, pp. 213–14.

93 Chinn, J. J., Martin, I. K., & Redmond, N. (2021) Health equity among black women in the United States. *Journal of Women's Health* 30(2): 212–19, p. 216.

94 Parker, G. (2020) *Restorative Yoga for Ethnic and Race-Based Stress and Trauma.* Singing Dragon.

95 Phillips, N., Park, I.-W., Robinson, J. R., & Jones, H. P. (2021) The perfect storm: COVID-19 health disparities in US blacks. *Journal of Racial and Ethnic Health Disparities* 8(5): 1153–60.

96 Phillips, N., Park, I.-W., Robinson, J. R., & Jones, H. P. (2021) The perfect storm: COVID-19 health disparities in US blacks. *Journal of Racial and Ethnic Health Disparities* 8(5): 1153–60.

97 Brewster, F. (2019) *Archetypal Grief: Slavery's Legacy of Intergenerational Child Loss.* Routledge.

98 Brewster, F. (2019) *Archetypal Grief: Slavery's Legacy of Intergenerational Child Loss.* Routledge, p. 115.

99 Brewster, F. (2020) *The Racial Complex: A Jungian Perspective on Culture and Race.* Routledge.

100 Brewster, F. (2020) *The Racial Complex: A Jungian Perspective on Culture and Race.* Routledge, p. 138.

101 Banaji, M. R., Fiske, S. T., & Massey, D. S. (2021) Systemic racism: individual and interactions, institutions and society. *Cognitive Research: Principles and Implications* 6: 82, p. 18.

102 Bock, B. C., Thind, H., Fava, J. L., Dunsiger, S., *et al.* (2019) Feasibility of yoga as a complementary therapy for patients with type 2 diabetes: The Healthy Active and in Control (HAiC) study. *Complementary Therapies in Medicine* 42: 125–31.

103 Rioux, J. & Howerter, A. (2019) Outcomes from a whole-systems ayurvedic medicine and yoga therapy treatment for obesity pilot study. *Journal of Alternative and Complementary Medicine* 25(Suppl. 1): S124–S137.

104 Basu-Ray, I., Metri, K., Khanra, D., Revankar, R., *et al.* (2022) A narrative review on yoga: a potential intervention for augmenting immunomodulation and mental health in COVID-19. *BMC Complementary Medicine and Therapies* 22(1): 191.

105 Green, C. R., Anderson, K. O., Baker, T. A., Campbell, L. C., *et al.* (2003) The unequal burden of pain: confronting racial and ethnic disparities in pain. *Pain Medicine* 4(3): 279

106 Nagendra H. R. (2020) Yoga for COVID-19. *International Journal of Yoga* 13(2): 87–8.

107 Weintraub, A. (2012) *Yoga Skills for Therapists: Effective Practices for Mood Management.* W. W. Norton, p. 19.

108 Raveendran, A. V., Deshpandae, A., & Joshi, S. R. (2018) Therapeutic role of yoga in type 2 diabetes. *Endocrinology and Metabolism (Seoul, Korea)* 33(3): 307–17.

109 Parker, G. (2020) *Restorative Yoga for Ethnic and Race-Based Stress and Trauma.* Singing Dragon, p. 48.

CHAPTER 7

1 Clarke, T. C., Barnes, P. M., Black L. I., Stussman, B. J., & Nahin, R.L. (2018) Use of Yoga, Meditation and Chiropractors among U.S. Adults Aged 18 and Over. Center for Disease Control and Prevention. National Center for Health Statistics Data Brief No. 325.

2 Morris, W. (Ed.) (1982) *The American Heritage Dictionary of the English Language: New College Edition.* Houghton Mifflin Company, p. 1484.

3 *The Holy Bible, English Standard Version* (2011) Crossway, Good News Publishers.

4   Feuerstein, G. (2001) *The Yoga Tradition: Its History, Literature, Philosophy and Practice*. Hohm Press, p. 6.

5   Feuerstein, G. (2001) *The Yoga Tradition: Its History, Literature, Philosophy and Practice*. Hohm Press, p. 215.

6   Pew Research Center (2014) *Religious Landscape Study*. www.pewresearch.org/religion/religious-landscape-study/racial-and-ethnic-composition/black.

7   Mamiya, L. (1999) The Black Church. In Appiah, K. A. & Gates Jr., H. L. (Eds.) *Africana: The Encyclopedia of the African and African American Experience*. Basic Civitas Books, p. 241.

8   Mamiya, L. (1999) The Black Church. In Appiah, K. A. & Gates Jr., H. L. (Eds.) *Africana: The Encyclopedia of the African and African American Experience*. Basic Civitas Books, p. 242.

9   DeShay, A. (n.d.) *The Black Church: Black Religious Statistics*. BlackDemographics. https://blackdemographics.com/culture/religion.

10 Said, O. (1831) *Oh ye Americans: the autobiography of Omar ibn Said an enslaved Muslim in the United States, 1831. The Making of African American Identity: Vol. I, 1500–1865*. National Humanities Center Resource Toolbox.

11 Said, O. (1831) *Oh ye Americans: the autobiography of Omar ibn Said an enslaved Muslim in the United States, 1831. The Making of African American Identity: Vol. I, 1500–1865*. National Humanities Center Resource Toolbox.

12 Goettner-Abendroth, H. (Ed.) (2009) *Societies of Peace: Matriarchies Past, Present and Future*. Inanna Publications & Education, p. 2.

13 Dorikon, W. J. (2009) Female Leadership among the Asante. In Goettner-Abendroth, H. (Ed.) *Societies of Peace: Matriarchies Past, Present and Future*. Inanna Publications & Education, pp. 117–28.

14 Keller, C. (2009) The Practice of Medicine in Matriarchal Societies. In Goettner-Abendroth, H. (Ed.) *Societies of Peace: Matriarchies Past, Present and Future*. Inanna Publications & Education, pp. 137–44.

15 Campbell, A. W. (n.d.) *The United Order of Tents*. Virginia Commonwealth University Libraries Social Welfare History Project. https://socialwelfare.library.vcu.edu/religious/the-united-order-of-tents-of-j-r-giddings-and-jollife-union.

16 Campbell, A. W. (n.d.) *The United Order of Tents*. Virginia Commonwealth University Libraries Social Welfare History Project. https://socialwelfare.library.vcu.edu/religious/the-united-order-of-tents-of-j-r-giddings-and-jollife-union.

17 Greenridge, K. (2017) *Secrets of the South: A Weekend with the United Order of Tents, a Semi-Covert Organization of Black Women*. Lenny. https://web.archive.org/web/20171010202942/http://www.lennyletter.com/life/a1014/united-order-of-tents.

18 Campbell, A. W. (n.d.) *The United Order of Tents*. Virginia Commonwealth University Libraries Social Welfare History Project. https://socialwelfare.library.vcu.edu/religious/the-united-order-of-tents-of-j-r-giddings-and-jollife-union.

19 Greenridge, K. (2017) *Secrets of the South: A Weekend with the United Order of Tents, a Semi-Covert Organization of Black Women*. Lenny. https://web.archive.org/web/20171010202942/http://www.lennyletter.com/life/a1014/united-order-of-tents.

20 Greenridge, K. (2017) *Secrets of the South: A Weekend with the United Order of Tents, a Semi-Covert Organization of Black Women*. Lenny. https://web.archive.org/web/20171010202942/http://www.lennyletter.com/life/a1014/united-order-of-tents.

21 Cone, J. H. (2020) *A Black Theology of Liberation: 50th Anniversary Edition*. Orbis Books, p. xxix.

22 Cone, J. H. (2020) *A Black Theology of Liberation: 50th Anniversary Edition*. Orbis Books, p. 5.

23 Cone, J. H. (2020) *A Black Theology of Liberation: 50th Anniversary Edition*. Orbis Books, p. 68.

24 Karenga, M. (n.d.) Bio Sketch. *Maulana Karenga.* https://maulanakarenga.org/bio-sketch.

25 Karenga, M. (n.d.) *Kwanzaa, a celebration of family, community and culture.* https://maulanakarenga.org/kwanzaa.

26 Karenga, M. (n.d.) *Kwanzaa, a celebration of family, community and culture.* https://maulanakarenga.org/kwanzaa.

27 Karenga, M. (2022, December 22) Kwanzaa, culture and the practice of freedom: a message and model for our times. *Los Angeles Sentinel,* p. C1.

28 Carrera, J. (2006) *Inside the Yoga Sutras: A Comprehensive Sourcebook for the Study and Practice of Patanjali's Yoga Sutras.* Integral Yoga Publications, p. 367.

CHAPTER 8

1 Library of Congress Copy Right Office (2012, June 22) *37 CFR Part 201. Registration of Claims to Copyright.* Federal Register. Vol. 77, No. 121. 37605.

2 Ranganathan, S. (2022) Yoga, the original philosophy: de-colonize your yoga therapy. *Yoga Therapy Today* (Winter): 32–7..

3 Lazarus, E. (1883, November 3) *The New Colossus.* National Park Service. Statue of Liberty. www.nps.gov/stli/learn/historyculture/colossus.htm#:~:text=%22Give%20me%20your%20tired%2C%20your,refuse%20of%20your%20teeming%20shore.

4 Jackson, L. M. (2019) *White Negroes: When Cornrows Were in Vogue...and Other Thoughts on Cultural Appropriation.* Beacon Press, p. 1.

5 Cherid, M. I. (2021) "Ain't got enough money to pay me respect": Blackfishing, cultural appropriation, and the commodification of Blackness. *Cultural Studies, Critical Methodologies* 21(5): 359–64.

6 Jackson, L. M. (2019) *White Negroes: When Cornrows Were in Vogue...and Other Thoughts on Cultural Appropriation.* Beacon Press, p. 4.

7 Jackson, L. M. (2019) *White Negroes: When Cornrows Were in Vogue...and Other Thoughts on Cultural Appropriation.* Beacon Press, p. 31.

8 Baitmangalkar, A. (n.d.) How we can work together to avoid cultural appropriation. *Yoga International.* https://yogainternational.com/article/view/how-we-can-work-together-to-avoid-cultural-appropriation-in-yoga.

CHAPTER 9

1 Yogapedia (2016) *Definition—What Does Lineage Mean?* Yogapedia. www.yogapedia.com/definition/4983/lineage#:~:text=In%20yoga%20terminology%2C%20lineage%20refers,the%20teachers%20that%20came%20before.

2 Vedanta is one of the six darshanas or Hindu philosophies. As one of the oldest philosophical schools, Vedanta follows the teachings of the Vedas, Upanishads, and Bhagavad Gita. Veda means "knowledge" and anta means "the end or goal of." It is the study of the search for the knowledge of God and the goal of the study of the Self.

3 Feuerstein, G. (2001) *The Yoga Tradition: Its History, Literature, Philosophy and Practice.* Hohm Press, p. 31.

4 Vedanta Society of New York (n.d.) *Swami Vivekanda.* www.vedantany.org/swami-vivekananda.

5 Self-Realization Fellowship (n.d.) Aims and ideals. Yogananda. https://yogananda.org/aims-and-ideals.

6 Self-Realization Fellowship (n.d.) Lineage and leadership. Yogananda. https://yogananda.org/lineage-and-leadership.

7   Self-Realization Fellowship (n.d.) *Paramahansa Yogananda*. Yogananda. https://yoganandasite.wordpress.com/2021/01/20/paramahansa-yoganandas-afro-american-yogoda-center-washington-d-c.

8   Self-Realization Fellowship (n.d.) Aims and ideals. Yogananda. https://yogananda.org/aims-and-ideals.

9   Heart of Yoga (n.d.) *T.K.V. Desikachar (1938–2016)*. www.heartofyoga.com/desikachar.

10 Iyengar, B.K.S. (1966/1979) *Light on Yoga, Revised Edition*. Schocken Books.

11 Iyengar, B.K.S. (1966/1979) *Light on Yoga, Revised Edition*. Schocken Books, p. 30.

12 Lasater, J. (1995) *Relax and Renew: Restful Yoga for Stressful Times*. Rodmell Press.

13 Kripalu Center for Yoga and Health (n.d.) *Our History*. Kripalu. https://kripalu.org/content/our-history.

14 Desai, K. (n.d.) *Biography*. kaminidesai. www.kaminidesai.com/biography.

15 Khalsa Healing Arts & Yoga Center (n.d.) *Yogi-Bajan*. Khalsahealing. https://khalsahealing.com/yogi-bhajan.

16 Khalsa Healing Arts & Yoga Center (n.d.) *Yogi-Bajan*. Khalsahealing. https://khalsahealing.com/yogi-bhajan.

17 Yoga Alliance (2020) *Our Standards*. Yogaalliance. www.yogaalliance.org/Our_Standards/The_Ethical_Commitment.

18 Baptiste, B. (2018, January 24). How Baron Baptiste grew up on yoga, & eventually got into the family business. *Yoga Journal*. www.yogajournal.com/lifestyle/balance/career/how-baron-baptiste-grew-up-on-yoga-got-into-the-family-business.

19 Powers, S. (2008) *Insight Yoga: An Innovative Synthesis of Traditional Yoga, Meditation and Eastern Approaches to Healing and Well-being*. Shambhala Press, p. 25.

20 Hotep, Y. R. (n.d.) Understanding the YogaSkills method and kemetic yoga: melding practice and philosophy. Kemeticyogaskills. https://kemeticyogaskills.com.

21 Ashby, S. M. (1995/2005) *Egyptian Yoga: The Philosophy of Enlightenment*. 10th Ed. Cruzian Mystic Books, p. 30.

22 Ashby, S. M. (1995/2005) *Egyptian Yoga: The Philosophy of Enlightenment*. 10th Ed. Cruzian Mystic Books, p. 29.

23 Bondy, D. (n.d.) The Black history of yoga: a short exploration of Kemetic Yoga. *Yoga International*. https://yogainternational.com/article/view/the-black-history-of-yoga, adapted from Bondy, D. & Heagberg, K. (2020) *Yoga Where You Are: Customize Your Practice for Your Body and Your Life*. Shambhala Publications.

24 Ashby, S. M. (1995/2005) *Egyptian Yoga: The Philosophy of Enlightenment*. 10th Ed. Cruzian Mystic Books, p. 27.

CHAPTER 10

1   Hamer, F. L. (1964, December 20) I'm sick and tired of being sick and tired. Iowa State University. https://awpc.cattcenter.iastate.edu/2019/08/09/im-sick-and-tired-of-being-sick-and-tired-dec-20-1964.

2   *The Holy Bible, English Standard Version (ESV)* (2001) Crossway, Good News Publishers.

3   Yoga Alliance (2020) *Our Standards*. Yogaalliance. www.yogaalliance.org/Our_Standards/The_Ethical_Commitment.

4   Parker, G. (2020) *Restorative Yoga for Ethnic and Race-Based Stress and Trauma*. Singing Dragon, p. 30.

5   Whitfield, C. T. (2020, July 27) Black yoga collectives aim to make space for healing. *New York Times*.

6   Whitfield, C. T. (2020, July 27) Black yoga collectives aim to make space for healing. *New York Times*.

7   Carrera, J. (2006) Glossary of Sanskrit terms. In *Inside the Yoga Sutras: A Comprehensive Sourcebook for the Study and Practice of Patanjali's Yoga Sutras*. Integral Yoga Publications, p. 369.

8   *The Holy Bible, English Standard Version (ESV)* (2001) Crossway, Good News Publishers.

9   Boon, B. (2007) Introduction in *Holy Yoga: Exercise for the Christian Body and Soul*. Holy Yoga Living.

10 Karenga, M. (n.d.) *Kwanzaa, a celebration of family, community and culture*. https://maulanakarenga.org/kwanzaa.

11 Karenga, M. (n.d.) *Kwanzaa, a celebration of family, community and culture*. https://maulanakarenga.org/kwanzaa.

12 Muhammad, M. A. (1990) *The Religion of Islam*. Ahmadiyya Anjuman Isha'at Islam; *The Holy Qur'an* (2002) (M. M. Ali, Trans.) Ahmadiyya Anjuman Isha'at Islam.

PART IV

1   Khalsa, S.B.S., Cohen, L., McCall, T., & Telles, S. (2016) *The Principles and Practice of Yoga in Health Care*. Handspring Publishing, p. 6.

2   American Psychological Association (2014) More than a quarter of U.S. adults say they're so stressed they can't function. www.apa.org/news/press/releases/stress/2014/highlights.

3   American Psychological Association (2022, October 19) More than a quarter of U.S. adults say they're so stressed they can't function. www.apa.org/news/press/releases/stress/2014/highlights.

4   American Psychological Association (2022, October) Stress in America. www.apa.org/news/press/releases/stress/index.

5   LePage, J. & Aboim, L. (2020) *Yoga Toolbox Project for Teachers and Students*. Integrative Yoga. https://iytyogatherapy.com/product/1-toolbox.

CHAPTER 11

1   Stephens, M. (2010) *Teaching Yoga: Essential Foundations and Techniques*. North Atlantic Books, pp. 5–6.

2   Stephens, M. (2010) *Teaching Yoga: Essential Foundations and Techniques*. North Atlantic Books, p. 6.

3   Williams, A.K., Owens, L.R., & Syedullah, J. (2016) *Radical Dharma: Talking Race, Love, and Liberation*. North Atlantic Books, p. xiv.

4   Whitwell, M. (2004) *Yoga of Heart: The Healing Power of Intimate Connection*. Lantern Books, pp. 62–3.

5   Whitwell, M. (2004) *Yoga of Heart: The Healing Power of Intimate Connection*. Lantern Books, pp. 62–3.

6   National Institute of Mental Health (n.d.) *Caring for Your Mental Health*. www.nimh.nih.gov/health/topics/caring-for-your-mental-health.

CHAPTER 12

1   Stephens, M. (2010) *Teaching Yoga: Essential Foundations and Techniques*. North Atlantic Books, p. 237.

2   Brown, R. P. & Gerbarg, P. L. (2012) *The Healing Power of the Breath: Simple Techniques to Reduce Stress and Anxiety, Enhance Concentration, and Balance Your Emotions*. Shambhala, p. 2.

3   McCall, T. (2007) *Yoga as Medicine: The Yogic Prescription for Health and Healing*. Bantam Books, p. xix.

4   Farhi, D. (1996) *The Breathing Book: Good Health and Vitality through Essential Breath Work.* Henry Holt and Company.

5   Stephens, M. (2010) *Teaching Yoga: Essential Foundations and Techniques.* North Atlantic Books, p. 241.

CHAPTER 13

1   Farhi, D. & Stuart, L. (2017) *Pathways to a Centered Body.* Embodied Wisdom Publishing, p. 6.

2   Arora, l. (2019) *Yoga.* YogSadhna.

3   Arora, l. (2019) *Yoga.* YogSadhna, p. 177.

4   Arora, l. (2019) *Yoga.* YogSadhna, p. 177.

5   Farhi, D. & Stuart, L. (2017) *Pathways to a Centered Body.* Embodied Wisdom Publishing.

CHAPTER 14

1   Stephens, M. (2010) *Teaching Yoga: Essential Foundations and Techniques.* North Atlantic Books, p. 357.

2   Le Page, J. & Le Page, L. (2014) *Mudras: For Healing and Transformation.* Integrative Yoga Therapy.

3   Mesko, S. (2013) *Healing Mudras: Yoga for Your Hands, Mudra Hands.* Mudra Hands Publishing, p. 19.

4   Le Page, J. & Le Page, L. (2014) *Mudras: For Healing and Transformation.* Integrative Yoga Therapy.

CHAPTER 15

1   Khalsa, D.S.Y. & Stauth, C. (2001) *Meditation as Medicine: Activate the Power of Your Natural Healing Force.* Fireside.

2   Gladding, R. (2011) You are not your brain. *Psychology Today.* www.psychologytoday.com/us/blog/use-your-mind-change-your-brain/201106/you-are-not-your-brain.

3   Parker, G. (2020) *Restorative Yoga for Ethnic and Race-Based Stress and Trauma.* Singing Dragon.

4   Harrell, S. (2021) Contemplative practice, meditation, & mindfulness. www.the-soulfulnesscenter.com/post/meditationandmindfulness.

5   Black Yoga Teachers Alliance (n.d) *Yoga as a Peace Practice.* www.blackyogateachersalliance.org/yoga-as-a-peace-practice.

6   CMind (2021) *The Tree of Contemplative Practices* [illustration]. The Center for Contemplative Mind in Society. www.contemplativemind.org/practices/tree.

7   Walsh, R. (2000) *Essential Spirituality: The 7 Central Practices to Awaken Heart and Mind.* John Wiley & Sons.

8   Saraswati, S. (2015) *Yoga Nidra.* Yoga Publications Trust.

9   Miller, R. (2022) *Yoga Nidra: The iRest Meditative Practice for Deep Relaxation and Healing.* Sounds True, p. xix.

10 Stanley, T. (2021) *Radiant Rest: Yoga Nidra for Deep Relaxation and Awakened Clarity.* Shambhala, p. 3.

11 Desai, K. (2017) *Yoga Nidra: The Art of Transformational Sleep.* Lotus Press, p. 1.

Author Biographies

Charlene Marie Muhammad and Marilyn Peppers-Citizen are certified yoga therapists (C-IAYT) with a combined study and practice of yoga of 50-plus years. As wellness practitioners, Charlene and Marilyn use an integrative approach to physical, emotional, and spiritual support to mentor individuals on their journeys of aging well. Each has an extensive teaching and training practice, providing workshops and lectures at local, regional, and national venues.

A graduate of Cornell University, Charlene holds a master of science degree in herbal medicine. Marilyn is a retired Air Force Colonel and holds a PhD in Public Policy and a master's degree in business and National Resource Strategy.

Both Charlene and Marilyn serve on the Board of Directors of the Black Yoga Teachers Alliance.

Index